REGINA'S RECORD

REGINA'S RECORD

by

JAMES ANTHONY VAN AMBER

Best wishes Always
James Anthony Van Amber

AnSer House
of Marlow

aHm Publishing

First published in the United Kingdom in the year 2000 by
AnSer House of Marlow, Publishing
Courtyard Offices, 3 High Street, Marlow,
Buckinghamshire SL7 1AX.

All rights reserved.
No part of this publication may be reproduced, stored in a retrieval system, or transmitted in any form, or by any means: electronic, mechanical, photocopying or otherwise, except for review purposes, without the prior written consent of the publisher.

© 2000 *AnSer House of Marlow* (Publishing)

British Library Cataloguing in Publication Data.
A CIP record of this book is available on request from the British Library.

ISBN 0 9517341 8 0

Cover design by Java Designs, Minneapolis, USA
Editor: Elaine Sihera, Marlow, UK
Copy Editor: Kerry Hughes, Reading, UK

Printed in the United Kingdom by
WBC Book Manufacturers, Mid-Glamorgan, Wales

Thou lustful and stupid one,
thou lean sow famine stricken and most impure,
thou wrinkled beast, thou mangy beast,
thou beast of all beasts the most beastly.

Middle Age chant exorcising Demons

In memory of Regina Jane and Mary Francis

For my wife, Mary and
Roger and Gene Broughten

"Allegations concerning the quality of care provided to a deceased veteran have recently surfaced. Because of the disturbing nature of some of these allegations, the Acting Under Secretary for Health asked VA's Medical Inspector's Office to conduct an extensive review of the veteran's records. The Medical Inspector's Office also has arranged for a board-certified, non-VA psychiatrist to review these records and report on the nature and quality of the treatment received. Because of the volume of medical records compiled in this case, it is not possible at this time to establish a time frame for completion of this review."

Office of Congressional Affairs
September 9, 1994

"The thing you need to know about me is that I don't lie, cheat, or steal and I can honestly tell you that we're not going to push this into history. We're going to be honest and by law we must be honest because that's our job. We're going to have fifteen people working on it here in the central office. We're going to talk to the people who were there. We're going to have an independent assessment. Let me assure you again that we're going to get to the bottom of what happened and we're not going to leave you out in the dark."

Dr. Davis Jarvis
Acting Inspector General
October 10, 1994

"After a thorough review of the records by the Office of Medical Inspection for the VA, it has been determined that the patient's quality of care often times exceeded standards set even today."

Dr. Miles Williams
Under Secretary for Health
Executive Brief
August 14, 1995

CONTENTS

March 27, 1951	11
Temper Tantrums	23
The State Hospital	34
No Place for a Female Here	43
For No Apparent Reason	52
Assess for Lobectomy	61
Ice Picks	79
Photograph	96
Lipstick	101
Mary Jane Forbes	111
Forty Seven Days in August	123
The Pit	126
Satchel Paige and The Cuban All-Stars	135
Man on His Knees	154
Walter Reed Army Hospital	163
Like Mother, Like Son	171
Regina is Crying	186
"O Little Town of Bethlehem"	205
The Blue Cart	209
"I had the most wonderful time."	221
"Do I know you from somewhere?"	225
Special Purpose Report: *Regina Jane Van Amber*	236
Postscript	243
Appendix	254

March 27, 1951

Sunday noon, four months before my sixth birthday, Mother got after me for the second time. "Under the bed, Jimmy," my grandmother shouted. "Get-under-the-bed-now!"

I have no memory of the butter knife, how Mother clutched it, what it meant in her hand, how her eyes appeared when she dropped to her knees on the linoleum, lay flat on her belly sliding toward me below the spring coils, spilling the chipped porcelain muss pot, pushing aside boxes, sliding on dust and urine, frantic, yelling, "You little! You little!"

My fingers had been working the tune knob on our brown Sears Silvertone radio. A glass of milk near my elbow spilled to the floor when I turned for something. Mother gripped my throat, trap-squeezed my breath. Grandmother forced Mother's arm aside, allowed me one big gasp, chance enough to skedaddle under the bed and I mean in a hurry!

Mother's shouts behind that old knife have been spared from my mind by the confusion, I suppose, of the moment.

My grandfather, idle with age, moved as fast as he would ever move again, dragged Mother out by her wild ankles, twisted the dull blade from her hand, sat on the edge of the mattress, gagged and hacked and coughed, caught his breath through more coughs, got color back in his palsied face and coaxed me out when things settled. Mother stood weak with regret in the doorway, pressed her hands down her face, wept through guilt, saying, "I'm so sorry. I don't know what got into me. I don't know."

One year earlier, during a howling January white-out, she

had argued with her parents that taking me on a five-mile hike to visit her brother Marvin was no risk. "He'll be just fine!" she said. "He's my son. I know!"

"It was twenty below zero," my grandmother told me. "You couldn't see the mailbox. My word! We couldn't let her do that!"

There was one other incident near the house. Mother and Grandmother were washing clothes on the brown grass outside the porch kitchen and for some reason stepped inside. The wringer washer rumbled nearby. I maneuvered a red step stool under the rollers, tempted the wet spin with my jacket cuff which caught, pulling my arm inward toward my elbow bone, my shoulder bone, my life. I screamed. Mother bolted outside, fell to her knees, jerked apart the electrical cords. Her quick thinking saved me. She released me from the rollers, carried me inside to my army cot, rubbed my arm, sat near me until I slept. Whatever she said – words that would have soothed any child – is not in my memory.

My struggle with the wringer-washer and Mother's outward display of goodness, or any previous act of kindness, were buried when her hand clamped my throat over the spilt milk.

I wanted her gone.

Two days later, at 10:00 a.m., Tuesday, March 27, 1951, my grandparents and two uncles stood before Judge Roy Baderlund in the county courthouse in Alexandria, Minnesota. The hearing lasted less than twenty minutes. Mother sat quietly in the rear of the court while the judge quizzed the family. Marvin, the oldest of Mother's three brothers, recounted some few events over the past month: Regina had left a waitress job in a nearby town without telling anyone where she was going. She traveled to Billings, Montana and found work as a nurse aide at St. Vincent's hospital. A psychiatric patient she was escorting to dinner on the fourth floor ran from her side, vaulted through the glass of a nearby window and plunged to his death. A week later, she reported a dead man on the floor near his bed. She sent a letter home with a prediction that something unusually heinous was going to happen. "I've been blamed for things I didn't do."

What frightened the family most about that letter, Marvin explained to the judge, was a statement about her son. "Jimmy should be raised by my parents, but not as a Catholic". No one understood what she meant. She is Catholic, Marvin said. She's real religious. Her son was baptized Catholic.

One week following what Mother had said about the two deaths, she met a man in Livingston, Montana. He worked in Yellowstone National Park. She liked him. He said that he liked her. She told him her trouble being a single mother filled with fear. He urged her to go home. He told her that he would pay for the ticket. She didn't come home. Instead, she began a taxi ride back and forth between Livingston and Yellowstone National Park. She mentioned to the driver that on a street corner in downtown Livingston a man's voice reverberated in her mind and said, "Go. Stop. Wait. No." The utterance frightened her. She wasn't sure who it was, what to do, what to think, how to respond. This story perplexed the cabby. She insisted on staying in the car where it was safe. She sobbed. She ordered the driver back to Livingston. On the trip, she changed her mind, pleaded with the cabby to return to Yellowstone.

In Yellowstone, she demanded that he take her back to Livingston. What do you think I should do, she asked. I know how this must sound. In Livingston, the taxi driver angled to the curb, parked, told Mother to wait, hurried from the cab, made a quick call to the sheriff. The sheriff came, asked questions, careful, deliberate questions. What seems to be the trouble here, Miss? No, that doesn't sound right. Not to me, he said, and added more, telling her that she was unreasonable, hysterical, out of control then he took her to the county jail in Billings. No one knows what will happen in jail. "You'll be safe in jail," he told her. She was furious and frightened. "Why are you doing this? What have I done wrong?" The sheriff called back to Minnesota. He requested that her family come get her. Two days later Marvin and my grandmother arrived in Billings by train. They got Mother out of jail, calmed her, walked with her to the rooming house where she'd been living out her neatness, her quiet concern, told her things would be all right, better when she got home. Marvin helped pack her suitcases. Grandma walked to St. Vincent's hospital, went up to the fourth floor, asked the head nurse about the dead men. The nurse said that indeed a man had leaped to his death from a window, but Regina was not to blame. The nurse went on to say that no one else had died that same week or the next, and no one in recent memory had been found dead near his bed.

They boarded the midnight train east. Mother stared out the window into the passing night. She said she did not like the hospital where she had worked. She wasn't specific. She said she rarely talked with anyone in the rooming house, had made no friends except the nice man who worked in Yellowstone. The sheriff was detestable, she said. She hated jail. "Jail is terrible," she said. "What did I do? Nothing, that's what. Nothing."

Following her return she agreed to see a doctor in Alexandria. Marvin's wife, Digna, drove her to the appointment on Broadway Street. "She looked pale like she hadn't slept in a month," Digna said. Her eyes were like pewter. "She cried and didn't stop, couldn't stop. I felt so sorry for her."

Dr Mather, the physician who examined her, had no specific training in the diagnosis or treatment of anxiety or depression or any number of other female mental health issues, yet his conclusion that Mother was having a nervous breakdown seemed logical and therefore became an official medical and subsequent legal fact. The family supported this idea. They explained to the judge how demanding she had become lately, how frenzied, how she refused to listen to reason. No one knew what to do with her anymore. "She has a fit whenever you ask her to do the smallest thing," my grandfather said.

No one brought up a word about spilt milk, the butter knife, the mayhem inside the house. "We didn't need to say anything about that," my grandmother said later. "We said enough the way it was."

Mother was not represented by counsel. The judge questioned her. "Don't you think you could use some rest, Miss Van Amber?"

No one remembers her reaction. Was it yes? Was it no? What was it?

A courtroom clerk asked Mother's date of birth. Mother stood. "October Tenth, Nineteen Twenty-one!"

"She don't forget dates," Marvin said.

Baderlund was inquisitive. "Do you know the birth dates of your brothers and sisters?"

Mother responded. Each name followed by each date, one after another in an abrupt, decisive, calculated list. Perfect.

"She does know her numbers and dates real good," Grandma told the judge.

Judge Baderlund, a stout little man with an eighth grade education, ordered Mother home to wait for the authorities. "You'll need hospital rest," he said. "You'll feel better with rest."

The family filled out documents and left. Baderlund signed the order for Mother's indefinite commitment to the state asylum at Fergus Falls, Minnesota or "until which time a facility for female veterans could be found". There would be no review of his decision, no legal review of anyone's decision again.

Around two-thirty that same afternoon my secret wish for Mother to leave was carried out. A thin man in a white, wide brimmed hat, a white jacket draped like steel over his shoulder, got out of a black car at the end of our driveway, got out and got into our lives for five minutes without end, maybe less than five minutes, five endless minutes.

My mother's name is Regina. I called her. "Mommy" those early years, my grandmother told me. "She loved you, Jimmy," my grandmother said. "And when she brought you things you always bounced up and down and said, oh thank you, Mommy, thank you."
 We lived in the country. Not a farm, but a little house about a hundred yards north of a lake named Maple, and a quarter mile east of the three saloon village of Forada. Our place was known as the old creamery house. A suspicious fire during the Great Depression had gutted a small creamery cooperative a few yards south of the well pump. The creamery was never rebuilt. People came by and picked the best bricks to line a walkway or a flower-bed, hauled away cream cans, said it was too bad there wasn't money to start again. I inherited a playground of rubble, and the jealous benefit of a large cement cream can table, curious to Maple Lake tourists who stopped on occasion, believing the ruined building had once been a small church, the smooth table its altar. My grandfather cleaned fish on that table, beat bullheads with a ball-peen hammer, poked a rusty ice pick through their skulls, stuck them on a board, skinned them alive. My grandparents husked sweet corn on that table, washed the garden vegetables,

cleaned a carburetor, cut off gopher legs for bounty. It became my stage and my stagecoach – a place of importance; the best spot to watch the Soo Line's caboose rumble past the elevator on the west edge of our village, watch monster threshing machines spew steady streams of wheat shrouded in billows of dust rising. I danced for Mother up there when she came home, jumped up and down, twirled so dangerous near the edge, waved, said, "Look at me!" From there I see red-wing blackbirds balance on the tip of cattails in the slough, and waves tease the lake shore under a mighty high mountain of great thunderheads exploding puff after puff of dirty-white speared perfect with golden shafts of sun.

The justice of nature, I was convinced, had worked the world into what it was, and my life at the creamery house held each day accountable to itself.

The man comes, moving along the ruins to the well-pump, angling now across the yard toward commotion in our porch kitchen.

I watch him stride with purpose, wonder why he hadn't driven in and honked or waved like friends or relatives always do. I had not yet connected Mother's recent fury to the man or his purpose. No one explained what was going to happen. Perhaps no one could.

Ted, our landlord, had watched me that day when the folks went into town. He had led me outside a few minutes earlier – just before the man came. Ted owned the house, took us in when I was a baby and we had no money. He lived in two quiet rooms on one side of the house. We rented the tiny porch kitchen and a small bedroom that also served as our living room. One upstairs room was available for Mother whenever she wanted to come home, but I have no memory of her there.

Ted was a kind person and quiet, careful about things. He had slivers of gold in his teeth. He ate peanut butter and jelly sandwiches, washed it down with coffee. Peanut butter and jelly sandwiches were all he ever ate except once a month when Grandma baked rolls and baking powder biscuits. Ted showed me on the front path how to solve the mystery of tying my shoes. "Dis-way," he said, working the laces to a royal snugness. "And you try it den, Yimmy."

Behind the oak on the wooded ridge that separates our place from the slough, the man drew close, less than a few steps from where I am, crouched, hiding where Ted left me.

"She's - sah stubborn bull in dere, Yimmy," Ted had told me. "Better off here you know, now."

The tree – its exposed roots large enough to curl into – was my safety, then wasn't. The trunk blocked some of my view, then didn't. Suddenly, from the porch kitchen, came this low moaning like a wounded dog, then a spectacular shrieking wail, curious and frightening. Someone came out the screen door. I pressed my hands flat over my ears to the whine of the spring pulling it back to slam (something I always did in anticipation of the bang). Through finger spaces I peeked past one side of the oak. Mother was a few steps behind Grandma. Grandma was picking at her high blood pressure scabs without a tissue to dab the blood. Grandma's face appeared stretched, grim, full of worry, the loose flesh under her neck swinging like a rope.

"You don't need that," she told the man. "She's nervous is all."

"You'll have to come with me," the man said. Those words made me cold, and I remember them now still as one of the lingering horrors behind all my thoughts, the constant feeling of something nagging, something breathless about to surge with power enough to blind me, hunt me, destroy me in a confused, twisted kind of excited terror as if I'd been given the authority to force Mother's exit, and I was now and forever cursed to accept the guilt of what was set in irreversible motion, taking place because of me, in front of me, a lesson of something unspoken, something wrapped in fear and more fear.

Mother balked, then stepped from Grandma's protection into a sudden flurry of jerks and motions and bursts of words lost to me by sight of her dress rising to an umbrella as she turned toward the porch kitchen and, in a running spin, fell. The man pounced on her. There were grunts and whining yelps. What was happening had no end. Hands and arms were rapid through the air. Mother was on her back kicking like a scared swimmer. Then grandfather's voice, weak, frightened, powerless, cracking, and then stronger. Something like: "Hear, hear, hear! Say, say, say! Hold your horses. Behave there! Now just a minute! Now just a God damn minute!"

My breath is completely out of me. My crotch is hot with pee. My shivering, it seems, will not stop. I fold my arms tight to my stomach, bend to the roots, beg for the return of my breathing, captured, it seems, by something inches outside of me, withholding from me its importance, my penalty.

Mother's brilliant underpants showed shiny clips holding each of her brown leg veins in place. Her black hair was wild, twisted ugly, without sheen. The dead grass, wires and threads gave her a crown. A shoe lay on its side, off by itself, and no one cared to notice. Mother was lifted to her feet, stunned, twisted one way then the other. The jacket swallowed her tight to her neck, belted and buckled, tight as a corset. She has no arms (a shock to my eyes between finger spaces). Where are her arms? She is sobbing through tears, saying that she was very, very sorry, begged in squeaks and whimpers and whines that she was very, very sorry, for everyone to please, just please leave her alone, said there had been a mistake and she had changed her mind and wouldn't it be better if she stayed after all. I believed her. I could rush out and tell everyone how sorry I was for the problems I had caused. We've made a mistake. Let her stay.

The man and my grandfather (what is he doing?) left the yard with Mother between them. They made their way past the well pump toward the driveway, the edge of the ruins. I ran from the tree, held my jacket low to hide my shame, then followed Grandma's retreat to the house. She seemed to fall forward, weeping as she returned to her doubt and pain in the porch kitchen.

Then the stranger's voice called to me.

"Say! Be a good boy. Bring that shoe."

I picked up the shoe, trotted to catch them, tried to run faster but my legs felt uncertain, filled heavy with lead. I reached the well pump with thoughts about the man. He might snatch me, wrestle me to the ground, scoot me away too. I caught up and stayed behind a little pretending there was better than good inside me that I – a good little traitor of retrieval – was like the three monkeys, had seen nothing, knew nothing, could say nothing evil. Pure goodness with only one shoe. Kid-good with a purpose.

When we reached the car I stood near its running board, gave my mother's shoe to the man who surprised me with candy.

"Take it, sonny," he said. "She'll be back before you can say Jack Robinson."

Mother was in the back seat. I dared not look at her face for fear she was watching – might say I shouldn't accept candy, might say I was an evil little shit, undeserving, a good boy bad with the Dickens, the little God damn brat.

The car turned into our driveway, backed out, left. A dust trail billowed between fields until the car turned and disappeared then reappeared beyond the sweep of corn stubble north of our house. The candy was green, yellow and white coconut in a clear wrapper. The colors seemed important to remember. I parted the wrapper, slid one piece off the white holder, nibbled and said Jack Robinson three times. "Jack Robinson," I said. "Jack Rob–in–son. Jack Robin–son."

I took a shortcut down through the cracked clay ditch up to the garden, making my way from there back to the house, reminding myself what I'd been told about eating candy slow to make it last. I moved from the ditch along that end of the garden to the path that separated the garden from the north cornfield, one last way to see the car. The path along that side of the garden was near where grandfather hoed up stone mashers and arrowheads and scrapers he saved in a shoe box under the bed, smooth stone mashers bigger than his fist, and arrowheads, some smaller than the tip of his little finger, and scrapers still almost as sharp as hoe heads. He flicked off dirt with his bent thumb, rubbed the pieces clean on his pant leg, on his shirt sleeve, spitting on it, rubbing, holding each piece to the front of his nose. "Sioux camp," he said. "And nobody can tell me different."

The garden, dark and gray with muddy circles sunken from the drain of winter, revealed rows of shriveled weeds limp and dead. The rows and mud patch circles were unsafe yet I might step on them if I strayed from the path. The path was safe and dry and straight, cracked into a long narrow puzzle of dirt pieces like the ditch, only bigger and blacker with salt-white edges.

I saw the car again where I knew it should be, small now between thumb and finger as the dust trailed low like a yellow cloud held only for moments on that one long road leaving.

This was all before the hope of baseball, of course, when Mr. Henry Aaron was batting cross-handed, waiting too for the glory of spring and a chance at life with the Black Bears of Mobile – during those thrilling days of yesteryear when the

REGINA'S RECORD

Lone Ranger and Tonto were best of friends.

> *When admitted here she was properly oriented in all three spheres and there was no evidence of injury, drugs or alcohol. She was underweight, nervous, and anxious, and appeared mildly concerned and tense. She claims to have had unusual conversations over the telephone. She apparently is not very particular in regard to her dress or personal appearance. She is a person not insane, but thoroughly unable to handle her own affairs. She has neglected her work and has an exaggerated opinion of her abilities. She received Electro-Convulsive Therapy three times a week, but required more sedation and occasionally five ECTs a day after which she became more tractable. Her progress is fairly encouraging."*
>
> Fergus Falls State Hospital
Fergus Falls, Minnesota
June, 1951

Temper Tantrums

Near the middle of May 1951, over a month after her court ordered exit, there was indirect word of trouble from the State hospital. Inside the hilltop maze of aging three-story buildings, towers, and chimney stacks overlooking the town of Fergus Falls, Doctor W. L. Carbehl, superintendent, sent a memo to Anna Clapshaw, a social worker in Mother's home county. Carbehl wanted to begin a more severe course of "assaultive behavior modifications" on his only female veteran who apparently wasn't cooperating. He requested an immediate assessment of "the patient's past in order to gain insight into this veteran's social and family history". His request was the equivalent of a criminal rap sheet for unmarried, flighty women. More paperwork, more justification, and possibly more funding (the State paid one hundred dollars for each lobotomy performed).

Regina was allowed work in the hospital's garden, her only freedom. She pulled weeds, working her way between long rows under warm clouds, glad for the luxury of washing her hands in the clean dirt, her fingers alive in the soil, doing something, one good thing after another, moving on her knees to snatch wild growth from its shallow root.

What is this place? Who are those who watch aliens on this earth? Are we moving into the

> *edges of an outer dark? Is this a low mission of some high order, chosen with purpose? Are we to say something about it? What is the purpose of our fears, our nightmares, our screams? Why are we afraid of what we do not understand? Who is this thief who comes in the night, distraction of our dreams?*

In Alexandria, Clapshaw spoke with Regina's Central High School guidance counselor, Wallace Dougherty, who, not unlike the judge and the local doctor before him, did not hesitate in rendering his own strong psychological opinion. "She was either elated or depressed," Dougherty told the social worker. "She didn't graduate with her class. She failed Latin. We held her back another year until she could complete her studies. She was not a leader in any respect and did not participate in any school functions or extracurricular activities."

Clapshaw interviewed Art Kolar, the County Veterans Service Officer. In order for the VA to reimburse the state hospital after her commitment, Kolar had requested Regina's service records. He reviewed them openly with Clapshaw. There was difficulty, Kolar noted. During her basic training in Des Moines, she had checked into the infirmary complaining of nasal congestion. What was that all about? Four months later while on regular leave in Spokane she sought treatment for physical and mental exhaustion. Something odd about that. A few months later, near the end of the war, she was hospitalized briefly at Dibble General Hospital – her permanent duty base in Menlo Park. She reported to the physician-on-call that she was having trouble sleeping, and crying a lot. She had always been emotional, she informed the doctor there, and admitted to biting her finger-nails as a child.

"Schizophrenic reaction, moderate to severe," the Army Captain noted for the record. "Temper tantrums as a child," he added, "but these tantrums were overlooked by the family. Physical examination reveals ruptured hymen. No further information available. Recommend immediate discharge."

Kolar mentioned that two of Regina's six brothers and sisters, Carl and Noreen, had also served during the war and there were no apparent problems. Regina is the youngest girl in the family, Kolar said. Three older sisters, two older brothers, then Carl, the youngest. "Miss Van Amber has a young son," Kolar said. "I don't believe she is married."

Clapshaw arranged a meeting with the second oldest sister, Noreen, who confided that Regina sometimes seemed distant, but wasn't sure what that meant or what had brought on the nervous condition except lately she didn't want to be tied down. "She was always a little different," Noreen said. "She read a lot and kept to herself." But yes she did have temper tantrums when she didn't get her way. And yes she did bite her finger-nails. And yes she stared off into space sometimes. And no she didn't go to barn dances like the rest of us girls.

Clapshaw met with Regina's sister-in-law, Digna, and Angelica, the sister closest in age.

"She wanted better school clothes instead of hand-me-downs," Digna told Clapshaw.

"Her clothes were as good as any we had," Angelica argued.

"When she wanted something extra for her lunch pail her parents always told her that they couldn't afford it," Digna said.

"She got as good as anyone else," Angelica responded. "The folks didn't have money."

"The boys teased her all the time because she was so awfully shy," Digna said.

"We were all picked on," Angelica said. "Boys will be boys."

"They were mean to her," Digna said. "They called her names."

Angelica fumed about what Digna had said to Clapshaw. Digna said Angelica had been spoiled and always got what she wanted. Digna didn't like what Noreen had said either. Digna said neither of the sisters knew what they were talking about.

A little later, the disagreement about Regina festered and Digna accused Noreen of being insensitive and the two refused to speak to each other again, ever. Digna accused Angelica of acting mean and those two refused to speak to each other again, ever.

Less than an hour after Mother had chased me under the bed that Sunday, we were in the kitchen in Marvin and Digna's farm home – a mud-brown stucco place a few miles north of the creamery house. I didn't connect the first incident with our presence at my uncle's place. The sequence of events, at the time, were lost in the angry mess. But soon after I had slipped out from under the bed Mother's frustration continued, and she rushed out of the house, slammed the porch kitchen door, and began walking to her oldest brother's place. After some discussion about what to do, my grandparents and I got into the Ford, took off after her, caught up with her by a small cemetery near Union Lake. She refused to get into the car. "Leave me alone," she said. "I'm walking!" But what else did she say? And why was she going to her brother's place? No one seems to want to remember what she said.

We drove ahead to the farmhouse, waited near their garden for sight her in the distance then moved inside as if we were afraid of a storm and needed shelter. Marvin and his wife and their four children had just returned from church. Grandma explained to Marvin what had happened. "I'm worried sick," she said. "Regina is not in her right mind," she said. "What will happen if she takes Jimmy and just picks up and leaves."

Marvin wore tattered seed caps, torn bib overalls, torn shirts, ripped rubber boots, manure-caked and rank. To see him in his Sunday suit was almost comical. His face was stiff and red above his starched collar and made him appear boiled. The white crease on his upper forehead looked buffed and sickly without a cap, struck naked below dark hair which always had a wet, greasy look, combed straight back in thin sweaty strands. In a suit, his hands seemed embarrassed, worthless without a wrench or a hammer. He appeared forced to remain tense and polite like a child punished and made to stand in a corner.

That afternoon in the small kitchen my grandmother stood near the south window, watching, speaking about something or other with her oldest son. Uncle Marvin was a man I knew best by the stream of vile curses that came steady from inside the barn or the machine shed – the times he held squealing pigs under the weight of one knee, used his jack-knife and sliced off their balls, cursing their struggle, flinging the bloody strings against the calf pen boards where a horde of wild cats had a howling feast. Marvin stung each cuss word, attaching his rage and disgust to anything that didn't work, or wouldn't do what he wanted, finding fault in busted carburetors, flanges, broken belts, flat tires, anything animal or mechanical. He gave the word cocksucker a special wickedness – a guttural grunt, and his pause between cock and sucker made it sound as if a stake had been driven into his heart – a man impaled between two words.

An older cousin told me with certain confidence that Marvin's cussing resulted from Aunt Digna forcing him to become Lutheran and the Pope had personally banned him outright from any chance at purgatory or heaven. I believed that to be true, and besides, Marvin didn't own a John Deere tractor like all Catholic farmers I knew, and that important fact supported the evidence that he was a heathen. I also believed his coerced conversion freed him to do other things Catholics could not, like all the times he bent over with surprise farts in his children's faces, strutting away, silly, in a sort of comic book cartoon glee as everyone scrambled from the room like gagging mice.

When Mother walked into the yard that afternoon, flung wide the yard gate, charged into the house, Marvin was leaning over the sink. My grandparents, Aunt Digna, and my cousins avoided the scene by stepping around the corner into the small living room. Mother and Marvin were separated by the width of a narrow table. I was standing at one end for some reason. Marvin was plunging the sink-pump for a cup of water. Mother said something, but what? No one wants to recall what it was. "I don't remember exactly," they say. "She was mad about this or that. You know – she was having a nervous breakdown."

Marvin froze, slowed his motion to a stop, stared through the window without turning to face her as if he'd seen something outside that left him paralyzed and speechless.

But when Marvin did turn to face Mother that afternoon, turned to say what he wanted to say, he appeared stuck without words in a puffed expression that seemed to draw him out of his own face, out of his being – something so vile it had locked his jaw and the only choice left was the speckled dipper in his pithy hand which suddenly exploded water across the table into Mother's face. Then the cup flew, spun in tinny clanks across the linoleum. Then came his reach, his thick arm, his meat-hand flat-and-sweeping in a blur ending in a terrific "whack!"

"Jesus f----g Christ!" he shouted. "You know better than that!"

I was petrified.

Mother bent, held that side of her face, pressed at her wet forehead with her other hand, pushed water off her brow then released a stream of her own curses – a rapid, demonic spit of words, masculine and deep like a growling dog inside a culvert: "You son of a bitch! God damn you, Marvin! God damn you!" And then she fell into sobs. "Why? Why? Why?"

I don't remember leaving, but I remember wanting to. My cousins had run upstairs in fear and shock, crying. Mother, I'm told, grabbed my arm and we hurried outside to the car.

"Something has to be done," grandma repeated her fears to Marvin. "She can't control her temper. We've got to do something. What can we do? I'm worried, Marvin. Sick."

I have no memory of actually fearing my mother, but from that day onward I was always acutely aware of where Uncle Marvin was in any place, any room, at all times, wherever and whenever we happened to be together. And years later, I had this question for my uncle: "Did you poke her, Marvin?" Did you get sloshed, come over for a visit when she was in high school and no one else was around, and she was smiling at you when you came in, grinning in that shy way she had with dream in her eyes?

Ted, our landlord, had just come up from the outhouse when Anna Clapshaw parked her car along the creamery ruins. Johnny Ray, the Prince of Wails, was on the Silvertone. And Dinah Shore. And Perry Como. And Hank Williams. And the Lone Ranger and Tonto at 12:15 p.m.

Grandma was in the porch kitchen. Grandpa was there too,

in his rocker, maneuvering the coffee can with his boot before he released a line of brown translucent spit, talking on and on about age or life or politics or the weather or things no one paid much attention to. I'd been in bed for a few days sapped by measles, ordered not to scratch the tiny scabs dotting my skin.

Mother's blue suitcase – the one with white trim – was under my cot, a reliquary of her life before mine and after. The year before graduating high school she had completed the "Home Hygiene and Care of the Sick" course sponsored by the American National Red Cross, checked out books on nursing from the public library, helped at home by straightening the house, doing dishes. She hated doing dishes. There were high school certificates of perfect attendance, a certificate for excellence in shorthand, one for typing forty words per minute with less than two mistakes. Two years after I was born she traveled to Spokane with the idea to advance her life (and mine?), enrolled in Spokane Business College, was accepted into Alpha Iota Business Sorority, ate lunch with classmates by the Spokane River, graduated with high grades (with the exception of Record Filing, which she failed and had to repeat), made friends, sipped formal tea on linen table cloths, attended Mass daily. There are snapshots of her leaning happily on a girlfriend's shoulder in Yellowstone where she often traveled during breaks, pictures and postcards of places she'd seen in the Northwest, a newspaper photo of Market Street at midnight during the war ("I was here many times," she wrote), a Camay soap bar wrapper from the Hotel Palimor, a stub from the Woman's Service Dormitory and Lounge on Van Ness and Market, a news clipping of Audie Murphy, the most decorated soldier in US History, saluted by a row of brass as he stepped off an airplane. There was a paper napkin from the Club De Anza in Santa Cruz with the words "Richard Boone" scrawled in one corner. She typed her favorite poetry, *A Child's Garden of Verses*, into a manila book and wrote: "Robert Louis Stevenson is my favorite poet."

Her life inside the suitcase was a paper life foreign to me, a postcard life, letters-to-home life; a life of fading postmarks, and dark green stamps, and orange stamps; a life of small photographs and dark negatives that had to be held to a bare bulb – a wishful, forward looking life of three embroidered cloths with the outline "Home Sweet Home" partially stitched. There is an 1847 William Rogers silver plate setting for two wrapped inside a faded lifetime guarantee, a beaded handbag, a brass service medal in which a woman is holding a broken arrow. There is a sweet lock of her golden baby hair in an envelope – its edges aged to yellow– and three novels: *None So Blind*, *Always With Me* and *The Cardinal*.

Ted turned his back from the social worker's advance toward the house, lowered his head, then shivered his entire body, shivered his lean frame as if just now attempting to finish taking a leak, squirt out the last drip. Ted never failed to shake himself that way when someone he didn't know or hadn't seen for a while came into the yard.

In the porch kitchen Clapshaw sat on the red foot-stool, eased into her questions about the family, opened a folder, and began taking notes. I stayed in my cot, coaxed there by Grandma who said it wouldn't be but a while before they were finished and she would open the bedroom door again.

My grandparents were polite but cautious with answers they gave Clapshaw, and didn't say too much, but social workers either do nothing or everything and Clapshaw had been busy. During the conversation she locked onto a comment about past insanity in the family (Mother's great aunt died in the state hospital after being clubbed repeatedly by her husband before he had her committed). And there were more questions, subtle questions, nice questions, and then personal conclusions about temper tantrums, clothes, finger nail biting, bad grades in high school, not holding a steady job in one place, substandard living, who my father was, where he was, and why wasn't his name on my birth certificate? Clapshaw had been very busy. She produced documents my grandparents had not seen – six year old information from a St. Paul social worker – statements when I was born condemning Mother for not "breast feeding", statements about "seeing her father as more like a grandfather", refusing to consider a Catholic adoption agency while she stayed in the Home of the Good Shepherd in the Cities, refusing to cooperate with "those better aware of her plight", "seeing herself as someone much more important than she is" and "being controlled by the wishes of her mother", a woman with a "full IQ at 90". There were statements about my mother not having female friends, not attending barn dances like her older sisters, repeatedly leaving home, questions and statements and conclusions and more questions and more conclusions. Clapshaw even aged my mother eight years, listing her as a "thirty-eight year old unmarried woman".

My grandfather wanted to believe Clapshaw was simply doing her job, a nice person come for a visit one day to get things straight. Grandmother wasn't so sure.

Clapshaw had the advantage of someone already captured, guilty by court commitment.

Wallflower, ugly duckling, unreliable, elated, depressed, a social misfit – Clapshaw, who had not spoken with Mother, sent her accumulation to Dr. Carbehl and her summation was clear. My mother, in the eyes of all that has been learned and is accurate, was a flighty ex-WAC, anti-religious, unmarried, self-centered, hot tempered; a finger-nail biting, stubborn, older country whore who could not support herself or her child.

Clapshaw's words, more or less, would weave their way into Mother's files in summary after summary, assessment after assessment, conclusion, diagnosis, history, prognosis – everything important would become more important depending on which doctor, nurse, aide, student nurse, social worker redefined it with slightly different words here and there, more or less, and then more rather than less; words meaning the same thing, repeated *ad infinitum*. After all, Clapshaw could say then and now: Aren't these things true?

I have followed my grandparents into the garden. My hoe brings up none of the garden's ancient secrets. My grandfather says I must strike the earth with force, dig deep before signs of other lives are revealed through the stone shapes hidden there.

I ask questions about them – who they were and why they were here and where they went. "Savages," he said, "camped here and howled at the moon until someone chased them off and they went somewhere else."

At dusk we burn weeds in the old barrel near the garden's edge. Smoke and fire rise sparking into tiny beads brilliant only for a moment against the evening sky. I am thoughtless and content without vision of what tomorrow may bring except excitement and hope.

REGINA'S RECORD

The State Hospital

> *"All patients must drink lots of milk and eat lots of butter for their health and well being."*
>
>   W.L. Carbehl, Superintendent
>   Fergus Falls State Hospital

A few days after Anna Clapshaw filed her report with Superintendent Carbehl, in the hospital's main dining hall – a long, narrow room with Romanesque pillars and high ceilings echoing the rattle of food trays, where as many as six hundred patients ate starchy food laced with saltpeter, Regina spotted Willard Nelson, a former high school classmate working as a kitchen aide. Whether he'd already heard of her trouble isn't known, but she convinced him of the importance of a letter to her brother Edward, a letter she told Nelson that she didn't want read by ward staff. He agreed to mail the letter and mentioned the incident to Edward a few months later.

"Fergus Falls State Hospital
    May 28, 1951

Dear Edward,
    Please come and get me. I'm much better now and I don't need to be here. It's important, Edward. All I need is a relative to say I can go. This is not a good place. They don't

listen. They treat you like animals in here. They're doing things I don't want them to do. I'll do better at home. I promise. Please, please won't you come as soon as you can?
                                                            Sis"

The morning Edward received the letter he showed it to his wife Rita, and along with their four young children, the couple drove to the creamery house from their home in Benson forty miles south. I played with my cousins in the yard while my aunt and uncle spoke to my grandparents about the letter. Grandma felt it was too soon to get Regina, wasn't sure about the procedure to do that anyway, worried aloud again that Regina would be so angry with the family if she got out early that she would decide to leave and take me with her. My grandfather agreed and showed Edward a recent letter from the hospital which said that Regina was doing much better but the staff felt it was premature yet to release her. The letter seemed official. It had the doctor's signature.

Edward put the letter from Regina in his wallet, still unsure, he told his wife, about what should be done.

In early June, my grandparents sold the old Model A and bought Ted's '38 Ford after he pulled in the driveway with a new, slant-back Chevrolet that appeared bright blue, paint job by God. That same week my grandparents and I made the forty-five mile drive west to see my mother, to verify if the letter she had sent to Edward could be trusted and to see if things were better. Grandma drove while I sat in the front between them to avoid getting carsick. Along the route, Grandpa pointed out multiple white "X" signs where people had met their ends in car crashes. Grandma countered by reading aloud *Burma Shave* signs:

REGINA'S RECORD

> *"If you pass . . .*
> *upon a slope . . .*
> *be sure to have . . .*
> *a periscope.*
> *Burma Shave."*

In a parking lot outside a large yellow building cornered with a tower resembling a castle, also yellow, I sat with Grandpa on the car's running board. When he adjusted his cap, I adjusted mine. When he spit, I spit. When he folded his arms, I folded mine. When he took a pinch of snuff, I watched, reminded always of German chocolate cake.

The day was warm. The sun's rays revealed a surreal elegance through tree branches thick with leaves. Across the street was a cement drinking fountain near a perfect lawn and a perfect sidewalk. Parking lots, cars, trees, endless brown brick buildings – a place, a city it seemed to me, large and complex and friendly.

When Grandma finally came out she rushed to meet us, told me to hurry and look up at this one window, wave. "Do you see?" She knelt and pointed, directing my eyes over her arm. "There! Up there, Jimmy. No – in that window. There! Oh darn it! She's gone," Grandma said. "I wanted you to see her, but maybe she saw you."

"I think she's much better," Grandma said after we settled in the car. "They said she was much better. She didn't seem as nervous about things."

During the visit with Regina, Grandma had not brought up the letter or the visit by the social worker. Regina's eyes were full of hope, she said, and there was no need to upset what seemed to be going well.

❖

Carbehl, the hospital's chief administrator and only physician, had a policy. "No visiting on Sundays and Holidays or after 7:00 p.m. weekdays." He had initiated the policy as a way to keep the number of visits at a minimum, control who was coming and going, and why. He'd been at the hospital over forty years, insisted on protecting himself and his staff from time not well spent chasing down patients. Weekdays most patients' relatives or friends had work obligations. Saturday visits were no convenience. Many of his patients came from farms. Families lived some distance from the hospital. Regina's youngest brother, Carl, had come on a Saturday, driven a hundred miles, brought some of her things, only to be told she was too upset to see anyone.

Carbehl was a punctilious man – a clean and neat freak. He demanded an attitude of resolve and compliance and order, a man who – according to those who knew him – detested any sign of excessive emotions. He believed emotions were the root cause of the world's trouble. No one ever questioned his authority. No one questioned his lack of credentials as a "psychiatrist". He *was* the state hospital. But whatever he was or wasn't as a physician or an administrator, three months following Regina's admission and less than a week after he read Clapshaw's report, he diagnosed her as incompetent, a person "thoroughly unable to handle her own affairs".

Do incompetent people remember birthdays? Autistic references to days and dates or not, Mother had no trouble remembering mine and the birthday card was postmarked four days before the actual date to arrive on time. The only oddity about the card was that she signed it: "Lots of love, Regina" as if to suggest that her privilege of motherhood had been revoked. The next month Carbehl wrote that she was "severely regressed, almost mute," and yet she had no difficulty remembering Grandma's birthday, and in full fluid handwriting another card arrived, timed to the day, her last words home:

"*From Regina & love to you all.*"

The hospital's main lobby, visiting rooms, and staff offices, according to those who worked there, were immaculate. Carbehl's orders. Mother's ward, a three story, brown brick building near the rear of the hospital, was bleak, sparsely furnished, an almost colorless place with dark green walls and mud brown doors and high white ceilings aged from cigarette smoke mushrooming on the tin ceiling squares.

Regina stood by her bed at dusk, stared out the metal mesh window. Will Edward come? Surely he got the letter. Surely he won't forget. Rita will tell him to come get me. I could stay with them. Things will be better. Or maybe Edward with tell Carl. Someone has to come. They'll come. I know they'll come.

One morning, early, aides shook Regina from her sleep, from her hopes of sliding into the car with her brother, driving off the hill for home.

You have an appointment with the doctor, Miss Van Amber. He wants to see you now.

Carbehl banned Regina from the garden, kept her in lock-up, shocked her twenty-two times during July and the first part of August – explosions of 130 volt electricity and the immediate aftermath of Grand Mal seizures, one after another after another after another. How often the leather straps to hold her body in place were not properly adjusted isn't known, but near the end of August that first year, Regina's upper spine began an abnormal forward shift, lordotic, torqued tight and twisted from bony fusions and violent muscle contractions, from stunning volts of electricity that arched her strapped body in four second explosions, some longer, none shorter. Crushed teeth were common. Vertebral fractures, pelvic fractures, muscle tears, and jaw dislocations caused by the threshold of each convulsion happened with horrible frequency. Headaches for life were common. Migraines for life were common. Screams were mandatory.

The shift in Mother's spine forced her to walk in a half-sideways, slightly bent-over gait which, after she was transferred later to the VA along with her records, government nurses described variously as: *"a Parkinsonian gait"*. *"[She] walks like an old woman on her last leg"*, *"A strange walk almost sideways and bent over"*, *"She ambulates really funny"*.

By late Sunday night, February 1, 1952, eleven months and a few days from the date of her admission, over 15,000 volts of electricity had screamed through Regina's body. She had suffered 350 grand mal seizures. In September alone, Carbehl shocked her three times a day for 15 continuous days, and five times a day for one week. Three times a day! Five times a day! And no spinal X-rays to understand why she was walking tense, twisted in pain, bent. No X-rays to look for fractures. Not then. Not later. Never.

Early the next morning, Monday, February 2, 1952, Tom and Candace Styles, a newly married couple who had just started working at the hospital, escorted Regina out of the desperate wards in the women's section, walked with her through the labyrinth of gloomy hallways and darkened tunnels. "You're going to a veterans' hospital in Tomah, Wisconsin," they said. "It's all arranged."

She walked with a noticeable limp, her upper body at an angle like someone turned permanently sideways to get through a crowd; hunched a little, her feet in thick-stemmed heels. Each step on a swollen right foot brought a piercing pang sharp as the repeated poke of a hot darning needle – sharp enough to make her wish that something could replace walking. The young couple escorted her out into the frozen morning to a waiting '46 Ford. Tom Styles put her bag of things in the trunk along with a file folder of hospital summaries, the sedation kit which contained two needles, two vials of sodium amytal (a truth serum used as a muscle relaxer) and a strait-jacket. Regina would soon be a problem for someone else, human property of the United States of America, the first female veteran of World War II in the State, transferred to a federal institution – the first VA experimental ward for women.

Regina sat in the front seat. A large welt extended across the bridge of her nose, under her hazel eyes, across her upper cheekbone like the lower half of a yellow and purple mask, sore and puffy.

Frank Sinatra was on the radio. Tony Bennett. Kate Smith. Pattie Page dancing with her darling to the Tennessee Waltz – her favorite song.

After an hour's drive east on the same road she'd traveled eleven months earlier, Styles slowed to Alexandria's city limits, passing the fairgrounds where County Commissioners had welcomed returning war veterans with free admission cards. Regina had glued her card in a scrapbook before going off to college.

The threesome passed places she'd seen often on her train trips through that end of the town – the large white tanks of Williams Bros. Pipeline Company, Land O' Lakes creamery, the electric company churning its sludge into a nearby lake, the water tower, the old baseball park, and, in the distance, the high school of her failure and more failure, and one last glimpse down Broadway Street, eight miles from home and as close as she would ever again get to her trouble and her comfort, then one-hundred, three-hundred, five-hundred – Mars, Venus, Pluto – traveling from one hell unable to beckon the cosmic timing of instant death from a massive swerve by an oncoming truck, unable to cheat her final fate by the luck of a slippery curve in a rollover, traveling safe with the soothe swing of Benny Goodman, the Mills Brothers, Nat King Cole, Rosemary Clooney; moving through a rolling ease of silos and red barns and crusted snow fields blinded sharp to the eye by sunlight, riding from that one hell behind her toward the unknown of another.

The garden is frozen, snow packed and lifeless with rows peaked where brittle weeds have risen high before death. I move across the sunlit glare to the mail-box with little fear my boots will sink through the glazed crust. From that end of the garden I look north for the black car bringing her home. Cars come that way, then turn north or continue east. Sometimes they turn south along our road and I feel my heart flutter until the car turns east again toward the village or moves past me toward the lake-shore and I am disappointed again.

Grandma has canned what she could and stored potatoes and onions in the dirt cellar below Ted's part of the house. In the porch kitchen, we set up our card table next to the kerosene stove and we eat string beans and corn and sweet potatoes and peas. Canned peas are nothing compared to their sweet taste in the garden. Sometimes we eat squash. We eat dill pickles and I shiver and wag my tongue and my grandmother laughs. We eat liver with onions, fried potatoes with eggs, boiled potatoes with corn and chicken, string beans with blackened hamburger and crisp fried potatoes. We eat boiled carrots with pork chops and Grandma scolds Grandpa for eating the fat. "God dammit, I'm not going to live forever," he says. "Can't a man eat what he likes?"

Whatever we eat, it is always mixed with the thick smell of kerosene from the glass tank next to the card table.

When old Ted eats peanut butter and jelly sandwiches in his part of the house, the mixture oozes through the gold slivers in his teeth.

No Place For a Female Here

It was dusk when the black Chevy rumbled over frost heaves on the bumpy road into Tomah VA, a row of connected buildings that loom large behind a tree grove northeast of downtown. Styles was tired, anxious to check his quiet passenger into Admissions, start back, stay overnight maybe in St. Paul, engorge his new bride.

In the main lot they got out of the warm car, shivering from the sudden night cold. Styles took Regina's things from the trunk, and handed his wife the records as the three walked toward the first complex. Regina limped between the two, her upper face puffed worse with purple and yellow, still throbbing from the impact of someone's fist or foot. Candace Styles took Regina's arm as she hobbled up steps through the first double doors into a small, empty lobby. Tom Styles took off his hat, walked ahead, asked someone for directions to Admissions, and found the office just was down the hall.

The clerk was about to shut the Dutch doors and leave for the day when the young man approached, introduced himself.

"We're the ones brought the veteran from Fergus Falls State Hospital," Styles said. "Minnesota."

The clerk gathered his thoughts. "Yes," he said, "they called. Early this morning I think it was." He glanced over Styles' shoulder to the women. "Where is he?"

"Not a he," Styles said. "The dark haired woman next to my wife."

"A female?" A wave of concern clouded the clerk's face. "No place for a female here."

Styles was more than surprised. He looked back at his wife and shrugged. "I don't understand the mix-up," he said to the clerk. "Didn't the people back there give you her name?"

"No one said anything about a female veteran." The clerk leaned over his desk sorting through papers. "Here," he said. "R Von Ramberg something – Von Amberg?"

"That's not right." Styles corrected the clerk's mistake, scratched his forehead, looked to his wife again, then asked the clerk what he thought they should do.

"Never heard of any VA hospitals that admit females," the clerk answered. "Not in Wisconsin. That I know. Suppose I could make some calls."

"If you could do that," Styles said. "We're kind of stuck here with this."

The clerk arranged for food from the main chow hall. The three ate in the lobby while a janitor opened a small office just down the hall. The room had a desk, couch, and two chairs. Still no word about a place for Regina before the clerk left, but he promised an answer one way or another by morning. Tom Styles tried to make himself comfortable in the lobby, positioned himself to see the door where his wife and Regina would rest. Someone brought pillows and wool blankets. Word spread throughout the hospital about what was happening. Open ward patients wandered by, curious. Hospital workers getting off shifts came by, curious. Styles was too agitated for sleep. Angered by the mix-up that he was given the wrong information, he wondered if they would have to take her back to the state hospital. He was disturbed by the number of patients wandering around, looking.

Regina curled on the small couch in the room, her foot relieved some from the pressure of walking. Mrs. Styles had pushed the two chairs close, propped her feet.

"You could take me home," Regina whispered. "No one would know."

"Everything will be fine," Mrs. Styles said. "You sleep now."

Did my mother think of me? Did she see me in her anxious mind, see my face in quiet peace, grin through the still dark at my thick black hair poking at the room's chill from under my quilt, pray for me there on my cot, think of Grandma and Grandpa and old Ted in his part of the cold house together so far away from the night static in her radio dreams?

After the early rise, a tray of eggs and hard toast, and another wait for information, someone in Administration approached Tom Styles. "You folks are in luck. Only place in the country for females. North Chicago. Opened the unit last year, but no one told us."

The trip across Wisconsin was uneventful. Regina was quiet, stared out the window, rode easy with the car's motion. They stopped once around noon, ate, then drove toward northern Illinois, and finally into Waukeegan about mid-afternoon. Styles couldn't find Downey VA Hospital on the map. He drove through Waukeegan streets looking, finally stopped at a filling station where the attendant pointed him south half a mile to Downey.

The hospital's buildings were secured by an eight-foot chain-link fence, made three feet higher by barbed wire strands forming a V on top. Styles drove through the hospital's main gate, slowed to a stop next to the single-level brick security building. While Mrs. Styles went inside, asked directions, Regina surveyed the three story red brick colonial structures and the pond.

"Why don't you leave your wife here, and take me home," she asked Styles.

"No. I can't do that."

"Why can't you? Tell them she's the one. They don't care who they get. You could take me home. I don't like this place."

REGINA'S RECORD

"No," he repeated. "I can't do that. Everything will be fine."

Styles followed his wife's directions as they drove to a small parking lot near the rear of the hospital, stopped in front of Building 100, got out, took the things from the trunk, and went inside.

It is 3:00 p.m., Tuesday, February 3, 1952.

While the Styles waited with her things in the Admissions office, two male aides appeared, told Regina to come with them, walked with her down a short hallway where they disappeared around a corner.

"She pretended catatonia most of the trip," Styles wrote into the record.

"When she did talk she talked to my husband and spoke with him more than me," Candace wrote. "The rest of the time she stared out the window. We didn't know her back at the hospital. We don't know why she is limping and walking the way she is. We didn't have many problems with her on the trip. She ate well."

The office clerk took their statements and the other files, typed a list of her valuables. *"Check for $75.01, baptismal certificate, birth certificate, honorable discharge card, American Legion membership card, Social Security card, Alpha Iota sorority membership card, WAC Enlisted Reserve Corp. identification card, gold colored wrist watch with expansion band, gold 1940 class ring, gold carved band, gold ring with three stones, pair gold earrings with stones, carved sterling silver ring, silver colored necklace, one key ring with six keys."*

The clerk put her things in a long gray box, wrote her last name, first name, and middle initial in large letters on the outside, wrote her VA claim number below her name, and the building and ward to which she was assigned.

Her two young escorts from the state hospital left building

100, got back into their car, and drove to the main gate. Tom Styles mentioned what Regina had proposed a few minutes earlier. "Can you blame her," his wife said. "Can you really blame her?"

Regina and the aides had come up the steps to 125D on third floor. The thick wooden door, a small wire window about eye level, opens into a middle hallway of glazed green and dark floor tiles layered with wax. The hallway is permeated with an odor of stinging disinfectant mixed with a rush of stale cigarette smoke, stronger near the Day Room.

Ward procedure of signing Regina in at the nurses' station, making a brief assessment of her condition and discussing ward rules, was put aside when Nurse Hixel saw "the woman's level of agitation and discomfort". *"Patient was led directly to the Hydro room where we had a better look at an injury to the female's face".*

She was ordered to take off her clothes. She looked at the men present and refused. The men began stripping her. She struggled, pushed them away. Another aide joined them. Her first conflict in Downey, less than fifteen minutes after her arrival, had started, but finally she agreed to shower if the men turned their backs and stood near the door.

The injury to her face must have given depth to her hazel eyes; made them shockingly narrow, her skin and nose still pulsating with pain like her sore foot. But through the shame and struggle of her forced nakedness and the hot shower, the nurse and the aides saw other bruises.

Nurse Hixel returned to her station to call for the Officer of the Day.

Dr. Taylor Scorba, the neuropsychiatrist in charge of the female section, was the OD that day. Scorba was a Board certified psychiatrist, highly intelligent, a small man with a steady soft voice, deliberate, cautious, full head of thick brown hair, wire rimmed glasses. He made his way onto third

REGINA'S RECORD

floor and into Hydro where he assessed his new patient's condition.

> *"Facial contusions on nose, upper cheek bones. Multiple bruises across abdomen,"* Scorba scribbled. *"Bruises, some three or four days old across left and right buttock, large bruise on right arm, small bruise on left arm above the elbow, bruise on left shoulder, lower left shoulder, back of right calf, left knee, right foot, right big toe, blisters on both little toes."* Scorba added: *"White stretch marks noted for future reference to past obesity or pregnancy,"* and *"Schizophrenic reaction unclassified. Hgt. 5' 5", Wt. 125. Small breasts, genitalia normal, does not appear acutely ill, confused. Does not like to be touched. Says she hurts. Observe."*

Regina stepped from the shower stall, held a towel in front of her. "I want my son," she repeated to the nurse. "I need to go home."

One aide took down a sheet hanging from a nearby wall hook. He dunked it in a water trough and opened it wide like a cape. Regina saw his action and became frightened. The nurse and aides snatched her towel, closed in and held her wet naked frame steady, forced her arms to her sides, forced her legs together. The first aide spun the wet sheet around her, double wrapped it quick around her sore body, her bruises, her disbelief – wrapped it from her neck to her ankles like a second skin, tight. Regina was screaming.

We'redoingthisforyourowngoodthiswillcalmyouthiswillhelpyourelax.

They forced her off her feet, lifted her like a big sack to a flat bed slotted with drain holes, and held her there while, one after another, sheets were dunked into the water tank, wrung out then plopped in loose rolls on her ankles, shins, knees, thighs, mid-section, chest, neck – pushed down hard, packed and stuffed around her, and on her, and around her head and neck, and high on her forehead until she had all but disappeared under the wet weight.

She said no and repeated no, asked them to stop, pleaded. She couldn't know what they were doing or what it meant. She became hysterical without moving, fearful without the ability to act out – helpless, frightened, unable to shift, rise, twist away, move.

We'redoingthisforyourowngoodtohelpyoucalmyourself, youneedthistocalmyouhelpyoustaystillquitfightingit,relax, remaincalmstopshoutingsimmerdown.

Three hours later she was released from Wet Sheet Pack, told to shower again and towel off. The sheets were hung on wall hooks to drip-dry. She was ordered into pajamas, robe, and cotton slippers, then escorted down to the first floor chow hall where the rest of the ward patients had already begun their meal. The room confused her. Scenes from the ordeal at the state hospital replayed themselves perhaps and she became frightened again, wondering what was happening, why she had been put into wet sheets, why she was being ordered here, there. She tried to leave, limp away. The nurse and the two aides stopped her, rushed her as she hobbled out the door bent-over, sobbing, then hurried her away and back up to third floor where she was stripped again, spun into another wet sheet, restuffed under another pile of impossible clumps.

We're doing this for your own good. This will calm you. This will help you relax.

"She screamed again," Hixel noted, "and continued screaming on and off for several minutes."

REGINA'S RECORD

Regina spent six hours in Wet Sheet Pack that afternoon and missed her first meal in Downey. She was led to a bunk, and, with "some additional resistance to the hypodermic needle", given a shot of Sodium Amytal before lights out as a ceaseless moaning and mumbles and sobs rise among salad-prayers from a few other women, frightened, each hoping for the gift of decent sleep through a hundred fears that might enter the darkened bunk room. This day, this night, the next day, and the next night, nothing here. None of this will ever just leave, stop, end.

And the solace of her things, her rings, her necklace, her jingle-jangle, her life typed on small printed cards, none of it can move from its resting place to the comfort of her skin, her hand, and the watch, her Bulova in the storage box two floors below – its tiny glass dial void of light in the cardboard black, the once steady hands without purpose, its faint ticking heart stopped. Waiting for someone in the VA to pluck it out, rewind it, slip it on the wrist, walk away self-assured that no one would ever know.

The women's ward in North Chicago had been open less than a year, a quarter century before females would officially be eligible for admission to all VA hospitals, and with some few exceptions, five to ten years beyond that before it would become a reality. The idea was to attract new psychiatrists and physicians, help round out their resumés through the experience of working with women, research female patients in order to find out whether their presence would be acceptable in a completely male dominated system, and possibly experiment on new methods to better understand the ten dimensions of mental illness.

The VA knew that many of the first female patients admitted would move through the system quickly, and some would not. Each female veteran admitted was observed for two weeks on 125 D, the third floor closed ward, then transferred down to the open ward on the second floor. The ideal stay, according to the VA, was six to eight weeks before discharge.

Then came Regina.

For No Apparent Reason

The entryways and hallways in Downey are dark, dull, rundown, and filthy – allowed to remain in disrepair by a VA budget bragging about tax money better spent not on psychiatric hospitals or patients, but on general medical facilities. Hallways are glazed dirty-yellow from constant cigarette smoke, butts squashed to dot floors and corners where shoe traces have sloshed in snow and dirt leaving grimy puddles near those male vets who often take comfort on the floor.

In the center of the hospital grounds, at the lowest point in the terrain, the frozen pond surrounded by a few oak trees is easily visible, and beyond, other buildings appear no different from Building 100. There is no garden.

Ward 125-D

The third floor Day Room in the female section has an upright piano in one corner, and nearby a magazine rack where patients take their choice of the Saturday Evening Post and Reader's Digest along with other magazines two and three years old. Several wooden chairs and two davenports are in no particular arrangement other than for the convenience of the housekeeper's mop soaking up coffee spills or vomit, urine, blood. The furniture is old military surplus from the last war or the one before that. One of the four wooden card tables has the progress of a five hundred-piece puzzle on it. The others are in use for card playing, letters home, a game of checkers, or a craft.

Tall, multiple pane windows, screened on the outside with metal mesh, surround the Day Room on three sides, separated at the far end by the extension of a three-season porch, locked for the winter. Knee high sections of iron radiators follow the base of the walls, each section extending out about three feet, topped with pads. Below the nurses' station window is a full-size phonograph with a built-in radio, and directly across from the nurses' station, a small alcove has been arranged for, as one nurse wrote "private reflections". The alcove has a davenport, a second small radio atop a bookshelf and, what the staff called their "lover tweet" a canary in a cage.

Each patient receives a list of rules, along with blankets, linen, wash cloths, towels, and an admission kit that contains a toothbrush, toothpaste and other hygienic items.

Rules

Patients are responsible for making their bunks no later than 6:30 a.m. Nightstands and wall lockers must be kept in order. You are expected to be clean and appear presentable at all times. Apply lipstick and makeup following your morning shower. Do not leave personal items unattended in the wash room. Remember the Golden Rule. Do not take what does not belong to you. Letter writing is encouraged, but will be read by staff. Morning rounds are at 7:30 a.m. Please stand at the end of your respective bunks as the OD greets you. Answer all of his questions to the best of your ability. Meals are 6:30-7:00 a.m., 11:30 a.m. and 5:30 p.m. daily. Remember, we are all here to help you get well.

Female Section
Downey VA

> "Patient slept sound during night. Taken to X-ray this morning. She is limping. Both feet are swollen and discolored. Face is discolored on nose and below eyes. Chart notes that there are other multiple bruises. Is confused and talks about her son. She appears clean but is not neat. Her hair is disheveled, her lipstick is smeared, and her clothes are not properly buttoned. Will answer questions willingly this a.m, but does not volunteer information. She appears to be friendly toward personnel and other patients, Laura Denner, in particular. When asked for a description of her life in the 'other hospital' she frequently grimaced and blocked. She is pale and she doesn't appear to focus well when looking at things. Her lips appear to be crusted and very dry. She followed the suggestion given and went to the fountain for a drink."
>
> Lucy McCann, LPN

"I don't want to be put in those cold sheets again," she told Scorba.

He didn't answer. He held up the first card, an ink-blot test, and asked her to describe what she saw.

She leaned forward a little over the edge of his desk, focused on the blot, saw the crawling lines staring at her, then let out a sudden gasp. "My God!" Without warning she oozed down off her chair and lay face up on the floor, her body trembling slightly.

"Why are we doing that, Miss Van Amber?"

"My back! I get muscle spasms. It's nothing."

She got to her feet, turned her back to Scorba, looked out the window to the frozen pond, changed the subject. "Isn't there an air station nearby?"

"There might be," Scorba said. "Why do you ask?"

"Aren't they going to drop something?"

"I don't know. Do you think someone is going to drop something?"

"It's horrible," she trembled. "They're going to drop something and it's horrible."

Scorba was writing furiously.

"What do you think is going to be dropped?"

"Can I go now? I want to go."

During her first fourteen days on 125-D, she played checkers with the nurses, worked algebra problems, read the newspaper, played songs on the piano by ear, and teamed up with her friend Laura Denner to finish a puzzle. There were no more packs those first two full weeks. In occupational therapy she worked on making a leather key case, and on Mondays and Wednesdays in music therapy, she listened and danced with nurses to Glenn Miller, the Andrews Sisters, Harry James, Tommy Dorsey.

"I'm feeling much better," she told a student nurse. "I should be able to go home soon."

She started a letter to her mother and stopped after a few paragraphs telling the nurse, "I am not sure what to say right now."

In the first floor chow hall, "She ate well, her manners were good. She volunteered for kitchen cleanup," but was denied by Scorba until "further diagnosis and therapy could be established". The day after Mother's work denial, Scorba filed a progress report:

REGINA'S RECORD

"Patient has been seen daily, except weekends, for the past two weeks since admission. Usually has been observed to be seated at a table playing with puzzles. Has remained quiet, somewhat seclusive, communicates little but does respond to inquiries with autistic references. She has shown no tendency to agitation, over-activity, combativeness or poor cooperation, but repeatedly asks not to put her in those cold sheets again. Speaks often of her son. She is neatly dressed and passively cooperates for interviews and examination. States she is feeling well and has no complaints. Still exhibits poor orientation and has no plans for the future. While seated at the table near therapist, she suddenly trembled momentarily, but when asked what provoked this response did not reply and said she was all right. All of her bruises are healing well. The right toe, which apparently revealed a fracture on X-ray, shows a healing of the subungual hematoma and she is able to ambulate on it well without pain. Her nose bridge still reveals some discoloration. Fresh gauze and tape have been applied. The extensive hematoma of the buttocks has practically completely healed and patient reveals only residual trivial discoloration of all the extensive additional bruises she presented upon admission. Treat with firm kindness."

T. Scorba, MD

A tension was created between Laura Denner and Regina at

noon on Monday, the seventeenth of February, 1952. Ward staff were directed to deliberately promote tensions on closed wards in order to create an atmosphere of reward and punishment as a method to establish patient leaders for ward convenience and information. Passes and privileges were given out or withheld on that basis. Laura Denner perhaps warned Regina about the consequences of a protest, overstepping this boundary or that line, not cooperating, attempting to speak out about ward policy. Or maybe it was an argument over something insignificant, a mistake in communication, an odd look, an accidental moment where something was dropped or pushed and taken the wrong way – a molehill to a mountain in one instant. Or maybe it was nothing. But whatever it was their argument escalated until other patients complained to the nurse who immediately called Scorba. He arrived on the ward in time to see five aides surrounding Regina. She was standing at the far end of the Day Room near the piano. "God dammit," she said, "President Truman should know about this."

Scorba gave orders for her to be taken to Pack. When aides got their grips on Regina, she shouted: "Take your hands off me! Get away! Leave me alone! I'll get better on my own."

This time in Pack, while aides fought to remove her clothes, she dropped to the floor, crossed her legs, and folded her arms, shouting, "Leave me alone! Leave me alone!" But the five aides got hold of her arms and legs, stretched her to her feet, forced her to stand straight while they stripped her, wrapped her in the wet restraint sheet, then plopped her on the slotted bed before dumping the thick rolls of dripping sheets on top of her.

She was still in Pack two hours later during a shift change, and one of the aides who had just come on duty, William Williams, came into the Hydro room and stood near the Pack bed. "Are we feeling better now, Miss?"

REGINA'S RECORD

She stared at him from under the heap, her eyes struck with a sudden, inexplicable fear. "Get out!" she shouted, trying to twist her head away. "Get away from me!"

Williams told her to calm now, then retreated from the curses that by now had changed to screams. She screamed, Williams wrote in his progress report, "on and off for about ten minutes".

"You shouldn't call colored people bad names," the charge nurse scolded Regina as she was released from Pack to shower. "It's not nice."

The nurse immediately called for ward aides, including Williams, and they repacked her a second time for three more hours. After the second Pack, as soon as she moved into the Day Room, she saw two new patients, Black women, who had been transferred over from C ward. "Jesus Christ! More!" she shouted, then hurried past them to the far end of the Day Room where she turned, and shouted more obscenities.

> "Miss Van Amber's language is foul. Repacked this p.m. for third time. Chased colored patients into the outer hallway. Says she does not like them. In Pack she struggled, and was given Sodium Amytal to relax her. She later apologized for her actions and said, 'I don't know what got into me. I'm so sorry.'"

> "After morning chow this a.m, patient Helen Hubbard attacked Regina Van Amber in the Day Room on D ward. Miss Hubbard pulled patient Miss Van Amber to floor, grabbed her by the hair and began kicking her about back, face, neck and chest. Seen by Dr. Scorba. The incident resulted

when Miss Van Amber took a magazine from the table."

"After Miss Van Amber returned from Pack this p.m., for no apparent reason she was attacked by Francis Stevens who was pulling her across the floor by her feet."

"Miss Van Amber and Miss Elizabeth Herer were involved in an altercation over some Kleenex in the washroom at 6:10 p.m. Miss Van Amber received numerous scratches on her face. Dr. Morrison OD notified."

"At 7:30 in the Day Room, watching a movie, Regina Van Amber told Dorothy Gunderson that she was a murderer. Dorothy threw a small object in Regina's direction, not hitting her. Regina lunged at Dorothy. Dorothy kicked Regina who fell to the floor. Dorothy, who was in cuff restraints, then kicked Regina on the left side of her face and neck."

"Miss Van Amber was found on bathroom floor crying this evening. When asked why she was crying she stated she wanted to go home. With some struggle Sodium Amytal was administered for discomfort, and she was taken to Hydro for Pack."

REGINA'S RECORD

I like my school. We are all in one room. Karen Merlson is the other first grader and we are both in the first row. Someday, she said, we will both be in the last row where the eighth graders sit and we will know everything there is to know on this earth.

During our noon break one day, my teacher, Hattie McClellan, showed me this important place on the side of the front steps. Someone you know carved her name there. "Regina" it says.

Assess for Lobectomy

At 3:00 p.m. Helen Harder snatched a folding chair, wound up and lunged in one short half-swing sideways, slammed it square and mean, as hard and mean as she could into Regina's face, into her chest, whacked her backwards off her chair, sent her banging over the Day Room floor into the radiators where she struck the top of her head.

I get out of school at three o'clock, walk the road home through the village swinging my Lone Ranger and Tonto lunch pail, past the abandoned bank, the old post office, Novak's grocery store, the three bars, sometimes skipping across ice coated gravel safe with stories of Dick and Jane running. When I cross the ditch into the garden, I pick the same straight path and run toward the house. From there I no longer dream of looking north to see the car bringing her home. Grandmother said she was somewhere else now – far behind me beyond the trees and the Forada village, and my school, and the big slough and the elevator, past where rails meet and curve in the direction where they said she went, curve to a point in gleaming narrow, too far to think about walking to see her in the land they call Chicago.

In spring, after one of my uncles came and tilled the garden with his tractor, we dropped seeds in long tidy rows following string lines toward the ditch. Seeds looked the same to me, but Grandma said they are different if I looked close. "And don't you dare get any mixed up, Jimmy. Otherwise," she says, "we won't know where everything is supposed to be."

During those first weeks we waited for signs of growth in the garden, my grandparents received an important document from Downey. We had a dictionary, but Grandma said that she couldn't find the words above where they wanted her signature. To understand what she was signing she would drive into Alexandria and speak with Dr. Mather. When she returned she told my grandfather what the doctor has told her.

"It's experimentation," Mather had said. "But the one thing you don't want them to do is cut into your daughter's head."

Dr Mather's secretary typed in a row of Xs across the sentence that read. "Permission to remove brain tissue." The doctor signed the paper as a witness and my grandmother followed with her own signature. Grandma sent the paper back to North Chicago where the VA date-stamped it before sending it up to Scorba's office for his signature. Scorba noted what my grandmother had agreed to, and what she hadn't, but instead of signing his name he carefully slipped it into Regina's files.

Ward 125 D was aroused at 6:00 a.m. by a night staff anxious to finish their shift. Throughout the five buildings which made up the hospital's psychiatric wards aides finished all night cribbage games, snuffed out cigarettes, stretched, yawned, relieved themselves, then moved in pairs into each sleep area for morning wake-up. The women's section in Building 100 had twenty-five beds on the second floor, and twenty-five on third floor lock-up.

Regina wanted to sleep, stay safe perhaps in dreams of driftwood teasing the sandy shore in some quiet cove, sleep and dream of silky fabric flowing easily over her body, clean sheets and pillow cases, the pleasant scent of flowers from a crystal vase on an oak dresser, wanted to sleep and dream before the morning rush of dangerous thoughts pierced her mind one after another in streams of mass diffusions, impressions sometimes impossible to integrate, memories unorganized, ideas rambling out of control through flashing scenes of her three older sisters standing in the yard speaking to her in mocking unison: Why on earth do you read those stupid romance books, Regina?

Her father's face maybe melted before her eyes then joined then blurred into each of her sisters' faces, each face somehow with her mother's warm eyes. Sometimes it was her father speaking, and sometimes it was another voice she did not know – hollow and raspy and frightening – and the faces came closer in a sudden roar, rushing her to overwhelm the morning light, drown the rattle of keys as aides came quickly through the double doors, calling for wake up. "Be damn sure you stay away from those Niggers in the Army," her father reminded her when she came home on leave from basic. "I know about Niggers. They stink and they'll steal you blind."

It was a story her father had repeated all of her childhood – about the time he was in the Army stationed in Lytle, Georgia during the Spanish American War. His aunt had written to him, warned him to watch out for the "darkies".

This morning she felt her back jolt to a stiff arch, not on the bunk rising to meet another hopeless day like the others, but without explanation she found herself lying on the Day Room floor near the radiators, bouncing in place as if the floor was heaving from a localized, concentrated tremor and the continuous quaking was thrashing her about like a shaking doll in repeated spasms of jerky unstoppable motions, the wrath of some angry, unseen hand. Scorba was called to observe the phenomenon, noted that it was an apparent "cataleptic seizure considered a schizophrenic motor manifestation".

The ward staff had watched too, moved close as the seizure subsided. Nurse Markum, the RN, pricked Regina's arm with a shot of Sodium Amytal to keep her relaxed. Scorba ordered her to Hydro for Pack.

The swirling enemy was everywhere now. Multiple faces, grim, distorted, pale, fattened, thinned – a house of shifting mirrors. Aides lifted her erect. Fast motion, faces peeling, exposing primitive teeth and skulls with flesh absent to the bone. She reached out and clawed aide Smithson's nose, kicked aide Boa on her shin, screamed and did not stop screaming while five aides carried her (one for each limb, and one for her head?) to Hydro, stripped her, spun her into a wet sheet, and placed her on the Pack bed. Her screams had upset the entire ward. In Pack, the volume of her screaming increased, and when she stopped screaming, she looked up from under the wet lumps, shouted, "I hope you all get a venereal disease!"

Three hours later, a few minutes after she lined up for chow, she called one aide a "bad name" and was forced into Hydro again, stripped against her will again, wrapped and lugged and dumped and layered again with the wet sheets.

Packs lasted three hours. There was no way to move, nothing to lash out with except her eyelids, her jaw, her tongue, the words, a long, long scream.

Fifteen minutes after the second Pack had ended, less than two minutes from the time she had been released, she walked into the Day Room, picked up the nearest card table and tipped it over. The aides rushed her. For the third time she fought her way into Hydro.

Nine hours in Pack that day.

The next morning, after chow, aide Sistler approached to

request her participation in Music Therapy. She stood, took two steps toward Sistler, ripped the name-tag from his shirt pocket, flung it spinning across the floor, and shouted, "Leave me alone you son-of-a-bitch!"

The aides formed a half-circle to make their grab. She braced herself behind a folding chair and refused to release her grip. As the five struggled to get her off her feet, chair and all, she used the legs and frame as a weapon, held it to her stomach, then poked and swung and pushed it at the aides – all the while suspended, carried by her feet and armpits the length of the Day Room, down the hall and into Hydro.

In her struggle to avoid Pack that morning, she bit down on her tongue and was bleeding "spontaneously from her mouth". There were two more Packs that day, and four pricks of Sodium Amytal, and two more Packs the next day, and four pricks of Sodium Amytal, three more Packs the next day, and shots, and Pack the next day – twice – and shots, and three Packs the next, and shots, and the next, and the next, and the next.

My grandmother told me that Regina was terrified of needles and did not like sleeping on her back.

Near the middle of March, Scorba spoke with Dr. Manley Morrison, and two psychologists. The four concluded a diagnosis of "Schizophrenia, hebephrenic type". "Hebe" in Hebrew meaning "young" or "youth", with Greek adding the "phren" or "mind". The four set a plan for the "assaultive therapies" to "modify her behavior" disregarding what was known five years earlier when the VA issued its 1947 "technical bulletin" which stated that electric shock therapy had no effect upon schizophrenic illnesses of more than two years duration. "The schizophrenic personality is not altered by electric shock therapy. Hebephrenics do not respond well to electric shock."

> "Followed Dr. Scorba and mimicked him as he made rounds. Doesn't want to be touched by aides and becomes agitated and suspicious when anyone approaches her. Her language remains foul."
>
> Lucy McCann, LPN

> "Patients Dorothy Gunderson and Louise Hansen both stated they would kill Regina Van Amber. When taken to Hydro [she] grabbed decks of cards off table and threw them at nurse, those attacking her, and other hospital aides. Caused several superficial bruises on Aide Sistler and Nurse La Roche."
>
> Nancy Becker, Student Nurse

> "Her topic this a.m. was about the government 'forcing everybody'. When aides took her to Hydro she resented heir holding her. 'Why are you always forcing me?'"
>
> Nancy Brenn, Nurse Aide

> "Had to be restrained before her medication could be administered this p.m. She scratched, kicked, attempted to bite and tore the buttons and part of a pocket from one of the aide's uniforms. Shouted many obscene and vulgar terms at aides. Taken to Hydro for Pack."
>
> Lucinda Cloaning, SN

Another fight took place the first afternoon Regina was allowed off the ward to go with a group to the canteen on the lower level. She'd been in Downey VA two months. Early that same morning she had followed Dr. Scorba around the ward and, for the second time in a week, mimicked him as he spoke with the other patients. How are we feeling this morning, Miss Hubbard? How are you this morning, Miss Hubbard, Miss Bird Brain? Are we feeling well? Are we feeling well, stupid?

Apparently Scorba had heard it all before. No Pack was ordered that morning, and only one hypo of Sodium Amytal about mid-morning for "agitation". Scorba even gave his permission to allow her off the ward around mid-afternoon. She took advantage of the coupon book she'd been handed and, in the small canteen bought a jar of face cream and a packet of bobby pins. After returning to the ward she took her things into the night quarters to put them away. Clarence Dominic, an aide, saw what was in her hand and pointed it out to the charge nurse.

Janice Tiel, a nursing student who observed what was happening, thought the aide wanted the cold cream jar to prevent breakage if something happened. Tiel didn't know that the nurse and ward aide couldn't have cared less about the cold cream jar. They wanted the bobby pins. Scorba had scheduled Regina for Shock the next morning.

Her initial resistance brought three aides from second floor to assist the four already trying to seize the bobby pins. She fought from the bunk area past the nurses' station into the Day Room's alcove, and finally into the Day Room. Patients scattered, shouting. The nurse hurried to get the hypodermic needle. Chairs and tables were knocked over, sent crashing across the floor. The magazine rack was tipped on its side. Regina ran, turned, ducked, pushed, hit, bit, scratched, kicked, shouted, fought off her attackers for almost ten minutes, refusing to surrender her bobby pins. She fought on her feet with her back to the wall, with her back on the floor, somehow got free to continue her fight behind the davenport, and on one side of the piano. When it was over, forced into submission by seven aides and a triple dose of Sodium Amytal still stinging her arm, she loosened her grip on the bobby pins, and fell to the floor.

The fight cost her three hours in Pack. When she was released, *"while putting her clothes back on in the Hydro room [she] slapped aide Williams on his face and was repacked"*.

She awoke to the prick of a nurse's needle and five aides surrounding her bunk. Sodium Amytal reduced her power to resist, not enough to stop her from kicking the nearest aide in the groin.

The shock room is small, with standing room for no more than Scorba, a nurse, and one aide – the prone patient on a narrow wooden table which stands about waist high. The shock table has a hump near its center. The hump is a sand-bag covered by a rubber sheet. The rubber sheet is covered by two regular sheets. Housekeeping will come in sooner or later and pick up the top sheets which have collected urine and the explosion of feces released between convulsions.

Regina's middle back is positioned on the sand-bag to avoid spinal injury as her body reacted to the violence. The nurse shoves one pillow under her buttocks and one under her legs. Pelvic fractures were common. The table has two leather restraint straps on each side near the hands and feet. Metal buckles are affixed outside each strap to prevent current from escaping the body, burning into the skin. A thick leather belt secured under the table is strapped over her stomach. Her hands are forced to her side, buckled loosely in the leather. Her legs are apart, also drawn loosely like her wrists and ankles, loose enough to allow for the extreme hyperextension, the suspension of her body in extreme rigidity. She is screaming. The gray, metal transformer plugged into the wall sits on a small table near Scorba's right hand. The timer-knob is set on four seconds. The voltmeter dial is set to 140 volts, 40 volts higher than the standard recommended voltage for women. Scorba not only disregarded other VA policies, but specific warnings to avoid EST when patients were hyperactive. Regina is thrashing in place, twisting to work free, cursing the day she was born.

Stay still. Relax.

Regina's heart is pounding. She knows what is happening.

The nurse swabbed a clear gel on each side of her temples, snapped a thick rubber band around her head above her eyebrows, and slid a two-inch metal electrode under the wide rubber just above each ear. They worked quickly, methodically, hurrying toward the knowledge that soon the savage screams, the protest, the struggle would stop. The nurse carefully and quickly inserted a blond rubber mouthpiece between Regina's teeth. The mouthpiece had a blond, four-inch air hole extension resembling the outer skin of an erect, uncircumcised penis. The aide positioned himself at the head of the table behind her head, prepared to grab her jaw to prevent a dislocation. She felt a second sudden prick on her arm, continued to scream. The nurse had stuck her with another hypo of Sodium Amytal to "enhance the convulsion".

The power of two baseball bats cracked each side of her head, snapped her spine stiff to an arch. The timer hummed to its first click. She felt the current.

  One Thousand One.

  One Thousand Two.

REGINA'S RECORD

One Thousand Three.
One Thousand Four.

Her body exploded to the restraints with force enough to cause deep red lines across her belly and each of her limbs. Her spine torqued tight, her neck muscles thickened, bulged – every muscle in her body burning, heated with current. Then came the first abrupt flexion. The Grand Mal jerked her body into an unstoppable series of violent, epileptic bounces. Then came the second flexion, as strong as the first, and the third and the fourth and the fifth and the sixth and the seventh and the eighth, ninth, tenth, eleventh, twelfth, thirteenth, fourteenth, fifteenth, and twenty-five more lasting a full forty seconds.

"Grand Mal achieved," the nurse jotted routinely on her chart.

Regina had lost consciousness.

Scorba put the head of his stethoscope on her sweaty chest, listened. The nurse pulled off the electrodes and rubber band, jerked free the mouthpiece, turned Regina's head to one side, then stuck a bent spoon inside her mouth to hold her tongue in place. The restraints were unbuckled. The aide stepped out into the hallway and lit a cigarette. Regina was still, her eyes closed, her tongue limp over the spoon. Her pajamas were soiled, soaking through to the pillow and sheet.

After the nurse checked her blood pressure, Scorba opened one eyelid and pointed his pen light into her pupil to determine the depth of her coma. Then Scorba and the nurse left. The aide stayed about thirty minutes until she came out of the stupor. She would be ordered to shower and change into regular clothes. If she didn't wake up during the thirty-minute time frame, give or take, the aide would get the nurse and the nurse would attempt to bring her around with oxygen or smelling salts. But her chest was rising and sinking, her black hair matted with sweat, her body limp with nothing but the deepest of nothingness.

Two hours later she was under the sheet rolls in Pack screaming. Packed again that day one hour later, and again around midnight. Nine hours.

The next morning the aides came again, and again she fought. The fight began in the sleep area, out the double doors, down the hall, and finally into the shock room. She did what she could to avoid her fate, defend her illness, her kaleidoscope of thoughts, her life. Each fight marked her body with one or two bruises, sometimes three or four, sometimes five or six. Quarter size welts on her legs, her arms, her back, her feet, her shoulders. And the next morning they came again, and the next, and the next. Each time she put up a vicious, fearful fight. Each time she screamed bloody fucking murder. Each fight was lost to the shock room.

And the next morning they came, and the next, and the next, and the next and two times more than the VA's own outdated number of not-more-than-twelve successive shock treatments. Fourteen Grand Mal seizures in fourteen days, and after the last, during knocked-out sleep, her ascension up carpeted steps to a throne, handmaids, court jesters, knights, bishops, the sparkle of fantastic jewels, glass slippers with a neat fit, soft velvet swishes from deep purple robes, a magnificent crown held ceremoniously above her head, held there for a moment, set in place then, adjusted, and, by unanimous proclamation, by right of birth, by everything pious and good, crowned above the squalor, coiled shit on the floor, puke, urine, blood. Yes, she rose above her own screams, above the belligerency of voices calling her from caverns: Cat-licker! Mother-fucker, whore, bitch, Mackerel-Snapper! And she rose then from her throne, greeted her subjects, the masses, the world, announced herself to the ward and the staff as the

REGINA'S RECORD

new Queen Elizabeth of England.

"Curtsey," she said when anyone came near. "Or else."

Within the week Scorba noted that the ward-staff was patronizing Regina, saw it as unprofessional, and vowed to do something. In mid-April, a week after the conclusion of the first course of ESTs, he ordered Coma Shock.

Her reign as Queen Elizabeth of ward 125 D would last exactly ninety-five days days, ninety-four of which were fought to avoid a room next to the shock room. It was no coincidence that the two rooms were close, but the reason was old, like everything else in the VA arsenal of attempting to control my mother. The shock table and shock box could be moved quickly from the EST room into the Insulin Coma Therapy room, set up, plugged in. The use of "Electro-Narcosis" with straight Insulin Induced Comas, like the other "treatments", was outdated. "Electro-Narcosis" had been on its way out for at least five years, and no longer considered what the VA later described as "state-of-the-art treatment".

Regina was forced onto the shock bed, wrestled into restraints, drilled with a hypo of Insulin (Sulfur and Zinc protein induced Hypoglycemia which induced a coma that was believed to have profound effects on the central nervous system). While she was deep in Coma, Scorba stunned her unsuspecting body with 140 volts of electricity for five seconds. After thirty or forty seconds, when the Grand Mal subsided, Scorba checked her pupils to guess the depth of her Coma, wrote down the figure on his chart, then went to the canteen for coffee. She would remain in Coma for three and a half hours.

Regina was dropped into the coma pit ninety-four times, twenty-four times beyond the outdated suggested course of "60 IST treatments". Each coma was a little deeper. Three times during IST, Scorba shocked her with 140 volts, and boasted in writing about the small number of incidents where she had to be revived with 150 cc of milk or 150 cc of orange juice.

> *"Her Insulin Therapy doesn't seem to be helping much. She appears to be regressing and her behavior at times continues to be violent and resistive."*
> Georgia Teller, LPN

> *"Patient refused to go to bed in the Insulin Room for a.m. ICT [Insulin Coma Therapy]. Hostile to aides. Struck at aide. In an attempt to restrain her, she received a scratch on her nose."*
> Lauren MacMillan, LPN

> *"Patient passed out near nurses' station. Insulin reaction. Revived with 150 cc of milk."*
> Camille Weider, SN

> *"Miss Van Amber was found fainted in the bathroom on floor. Her pulse was thready. Insulin reaction. Revived and taken to bed."*
> Lauren MacMillan, LPN

> *"While in group going to physical therapy on lower level, Van Amber attempted to elope by north exit and ran outside toward the pond. Guards called and patient escorted back to ward. Refused explanation for her behavior saying, 'It's*

REGINA'S RECORD

none of your G-D business if I want to kill myself'. Following Pack, shouted continuously, from 5:30 until 5:45, the three words, 'Leave Me Alone'."

Mary Frederick, LPN

"Although Regina is a neat appearing girl, she walks with a definite stoop and an uncertain gait. Is very hostile towards all aides. They force me to do things, she says often."

Sally Diment, SN

"While seated in the Day Room, for no apparent reason, patient Dorothy Gunderson repeatedly slapped Regina. Miss Van Amber did not respond, but she is on a heavy dosage of Sodium Amytal this a.m. No apparent injuries."

Sally Diment, SN

Mrs. Doris Goldberg, a social worker, found Regina sitting near the radiators in the Day Room, approached with caution, asked if they could talk. "Curtsy first," she demanded. "I'm Elizabeth, Queen of England and if you don't know that you should."

Goldberg obliged with a curtsy, took a few steps closer, introduced herself.

"Permission to go with Your Highness downstairs to the chow hall. We can talk there."

Without protest Regina followed the social worker past the nurses' station to the hallway where Goldberg unlocked the door. They found the first floor chow hall empty and took a seat. The social worker explained that she wanted to find out more about Regina's past and asked if that was okay.

Regina nodded, her eyes distant, cloudy.

"You have a child, I understand."

"I had two children, I think, but I'm not married."

"Could you tell me about yourself? What you did before?"

"Why do you need to know this?"

"We're trying to understand you . . . to help you get better."

"I can't go home," she sobbed. "I can't. Don't you understand?"

"Could you tell me the names of your brothers and sisters?"

She recited the names, counting each on her fingers until she came to six.

"And me – that's seven," she said.

"How old is your son?"

"Six."

"Do you remember the name of the father of your child?"

"No."

"Is there anything you would like me to do?" Goldberg asked.

"Can we go now?" Regina stood, looked anxiously toward the door, then started to walk away.

"Could we talk again?" asked Goldberg as she stood to catch up. "I want to get to know you – hear more of your story."

"No one will ever tell my story."

> "At 2:30 p.m., it was noted that Pt. Regina Van Amber had several bruises on her left arm and both thighs. Pt. has been very combative and hyperactive requiring restraints and hydrotherapy [a tub of hot water covered with a rubber sheet and hole for the head], and sedative Packs. It is

usually necessary for 5 or 6 people to hold her in order to get her into restraint."

Nancy Brenn, NA

"The patient is very sarcastic and has a hostile and faraway look in her eyes. When taken to Pack, patient suddenly began fighting aides and other personnel, scratching, kicking – very hard to manage, taking 5 aides and 3 nurses to hold her while getting ready for Pack. During the struggle several bruises were sustained by the patient. Several aides were scratched. Remains belligerent in Pack."

Lucinda Cloaning, SN

"During altercation with Beatrice Wood by bunks this a.m., patient was thrown to the floor where she sustained an abrasion on back of right shoulder and reddened area on back. Taken to Pack."

Lauren MacMillan, LPN

"Patient found on floor in latrine crying. States that she's sorry she gets upset over things, said, 'Why don't they just leave me alone when I get like that?'"

Nancy Brenn, NA

Struggles to remove Mother's clothes in Hydro were not counted as assaultive, nor were the high number of incidents where the aides forced her against her will toward a specific "treatment module".

Nurses recorded 318 additional references to her being "combative, assaultive" and "resistive" in 1952, and 216 notations of being "fearful" or "markedly fearful" of Electric Shock, Insulin Coma, Sedative Pack, Hydrotherapy, needles, aides, and other patients. She was assaulted with chairs, kicked, slapped, beaten, and pulled across the floor by her hair.

She was poked with 302 hypos of Sodium Amytal that year. From mid-April to late August, Scorba dropped her into a coma a total of 282 hours. She spent 461 hours and thirty minutes in restraints (not counting Pack times) for periods of up to twenty-two hours per day. She struggled in full-bed restraints for twenty-four days out of thirty-one in August, and it was noted on sixteen occasions that she "begged" or "asked" or "pleaded" to go home. She "refused" food twenty-two times and "accepted orange juice" once. She missed 57 regular meals while stuffed under wet sheets, 128 meals while in restraint, and 83 meals deep in a coma.

She was "packed" 3 hours a day, 5 days a week for three continuous weeks in November 1952, and 3 hours a day for twenty-six continuous days in December. Twelve times she was packed for 9 hours, twice for 10, and once for 12 hours.

On Christmas Eve, *White Christmas*, Bing Crosby's greatest hit played on the Day Room radio. Just down the hall, Regina was laboring in her sixth hour wrapped under packed sheets. She weighed ninety-two pounds.

I got a Lone Ranger jackknife from my grandparents, Lincoln logs from Uncle Carl and Aunt Ellen, and a fifty-cent piece from Hattie McClellan, my teacher. Christmas morning someone left a box of gifts in the dead snow outside the porch kitchen. Grandma acted surprised to find it there, wondered out loud if we should keep the box. I told her we should not keep it. There had been a program on the Silvertone called "Jingle Bells" where this man introduced singers, begged for people to pledge money, and proclaimed that all poor people would get gifts for Christmas. My red Lone Ranger jackknife, the Lincoln Logs, and my fifty-cent piece gave me rights far above poverty, and, because Ted got nothing – holy and quiet in his part of the house – why not give the box to him? Grandma said that Ted didn't celebrate Christmas, and she put the box under the kerosene stove. Later, when I couldn't resist, we opened the packages. There was candy cane, a magic slate with a wood stick pencil (red), dominoes, a puzzle, a yo-yo, and a long string of what I later came to know was shame.

Two days after Christmas, inside Downey, Scorba and Morrison talked about Regina's case. Scorba jotted down the words: "Assess for Lobectomy."

In his final report on Regina's first eleven months in Downey VA, Scorba noted: *"At least we got her to stop saying she was Queen Elizabeth"*.

The following morning, New Year's eve, Regina approached the nurse's station where Morrison, who was OD that day, and Nurse Markum were standing, chatting.

"I am Queen Victoria," Regina announced, "and don't you people ever forget it!"

Ice Picks

> *"During altercation with Beatrice Wood by bunks this a.m, patient was thrown to the floor where she sustained an abrasion on back of right shoulder and reddened area on back. Taken to Pack."*
> Lauren MacMillan, LPN
> January 10, 1953

By the end of January, Regina, at five feet five inches tall was an eighty-five pound stick woman. Her mind was ordering her body to die, and her body was responding.

Scorba was aware that Insulin and Electric Shock, for reasons unclear, increased appetite. In Regina's case, none of the previous "therapies" had been effective for weight gain (or anything else), but Scorba decided to go again, decided on the Shock Box to avoid the risk of a permanent coma, and ordered another course of twelve ESTs on Regina. Once the Grand Mal seizures ceased and she regained consciousness, Scorba guessed that her food intake would increase and he wouldn't have to explain a thirty-two year old dead woman.

The predawn fights with aides shaking her from the comfort of sleep once again meant a body covered with scrapes, scratches, bumps and bruises.

"Her screaming and fighting and foul language," Nurse MacMillan said, "*is almost continuous prior to each EST. Numerous abrasions sustained by patient.*"

REGINA'S RECORD

In the shock room, Scorba cranked the voltage meter to 130 volts then blasted Regina's frail bones rigid and taut into the loose leather straps. Four long seconds suspended by the electric rocket machine.

Seventeen patients around the country had died from the effects of Electric Shock the year before. There may have been more. The VA claimed none of those deaths and shifted fault to state hospitals that had reported them. But the VA's Central Office, to justify their own use of shock, attributed those fatalities to other complications specifically: "Advanced syphilis, and pulmonary conditions not previously known".

Scorba continued to shock Regina, and the effect he was looking for followed the first EST. Regina ate like a starved animal. She even refused the restriction of utensils, stuffed food in her mouth, pushed scrambled eggs down her face to feel their warm wonder before shoving them between her lips, licking the tray, demanding more. She gulped milk, gulped hot coffee, gulped orange juice, devoured toast, ate food from other patients' trays, ate handfuls of butter, ate everything, and wanted more. She could not wait to eat. When she wasn't in Wet Sheet Pack or bed restraints, she was first in the chow line for breakfast, dinner, and supper. She fought her way to eat. Shoved other patients aside in order to eat. "Get out of my way," she said. "I'm going to eat!" Sometimes she ran ahead to make sure she got inside the chow hall well ahead of the others in order to load up her tray.

The staff, repulsed by her latest behavior over food, reported her "animalistic eating behavior" and Scorba promptly scheduled "Etiquette Therapy".

Regina was taken into a private room and, as two aides looked on, a woman from Occupational Therapy ordered her to sit behind a table. The woman laid out a place setting of flatware next to an empty tray, cup and saucer.

"Miss Van Amber," the woman began, "please pick up the fork with your right hand and ever so gently, like a lady, show us how you will eat your delicious meal."

"Where's the food?" Regina shouted, and with one arm swept the display off the table where it crashed to the floor. "I want food!"

> "This patient refused to cooperate in Etiquette Therapy! I cannot be expected to help this person when her table manners are so inappropriate. She does not follow instructions."
>
> Agnes Wallaby, OT

> "Miss Van Amber had an altercation with aides in Etiquette Therapy this p.m. Packed three hours. Sustained bruise on knee when slipping on [the] Hydro room floor following Pack. Said she doesn't hurt and to leave her alone. No other apparent injuries. Seen by Dr. Morrison."

Near the middle of February, after twelve successive shock treatments Regina weighed 130 pounds. Her belly was distended.

By the end of February she weighed 140 pounds.

Three weeks later she was at 160 pounds and her high energy level and continued resistance to Wet Sheet Pack and the hypodermic needle meant more of a sustained struggle with aides who now complained that she was even more difficult to manage.

Scorba put her on a special diet, but she continued to add pounds, then refused to step on the scale until aides forced her. Finally, a nurse and two aides approached her in the Day Room, stood back a few steps in case there was trouble, then told her directly that she needed to lose weight – that she was getting "very fat".

Regina stood, walked to the corner near the piano, and banged her head on the keys, weeping. "Put me in your sheets then," she sobbed. "Take me now. Put me in your sheets!"

> *"Sedative Pack 3 hrs this p.m. at her own request. Did ask aides not to touch her. Cooperated well."*

Maxwell Sirca, chief administrator at Downey, was eventually made aware of the trouble Regina had been causing since her admission and requested the first of two research studies to determine why the woman was so "markedly fearful and resistive to treatment". The research study was to be conducted by re-examining ward reports, progress notes, doctors orders, and other pertinent records that the staff in the Female Section had compiled. In addition, Sirca directed staff members on 125 D *"to observe Miss Van Amber in her present environment and make recommendations for future consideration"*.

One psychologist had suggested that Regina's violent behavior and resistive attitude was a post reaction to the "incestuous nature of the brother and sister relationship, and her thinking leaned toward male dominated roles". A second Downey psychologist supported that theory adding that family rejection had played a major role as well. "She sees herself as the ugly duckling".

On March 10, Regina was scheduled for a regular dental appointment. When aides gathered to escort her from the ward she refused, stood behind her chair ready for another fierce fight. The nursing staff quickly called off the aides – in order to avoid being named as a negative in the research study? – and her refusal was accepted without a struggle. Twice before she had refused to see the dentist, and twice fought with aides until nurses decided that the dentist wouldn't be able to perform his exam, anyway. After each refusal, the ward nurse had called and canceled the appointment due to her "level of agitation".

The dentist (who held office hours two days a week in another building) noted the date, time, and reason for the cancellation. Unlike the accumulation of progress notes and doctors orders that Scorba, Morrison and the nursing staff could access or review at will, Regina's dental chart was kept solely by the dentist in his office. That single page document remained apart from the possibility of any change or manipulation by the two physicians or anyone else on 125 D. More importantly, because of its separate location in the dentist's file cabinet, the record of when she was supposed to be there, and why she refused each appointment, remained intact.

It was the one document, a few months later which Morrison and Scorba either overlooked, or didn't consider important when they agreed to cover up an irreversible medical blunder.

The Lobotomy Staff met at noon on March 15. Scorba, Morrison, one psychologist, and the hospital's chief administrator, Maxwell Sirca, discussed Regina's case. The authorization form that my grandmother had signed and sent with Dr. Mather's restrictions had been disregarded. Morrison was against delaying any decision, but the majority vote was to meet again following skull X-rays, an EEG and blood work. The Lobotomy Staff would look for signs of brain deterioration, monitor her behavior through the research study and then make a final decision.

❖

REGINA'S RECORD

Near our bedroom window in Ted's place, Grandpa caught the heel of his boot on the edge of the linoleum. He fell with a tremendous thump, lay helpless on the floor, and groaned.

"What on earth, Ray!" Grandma rushed in from the porch kitchen, gasped, tried to help him up.

"My hip," he moaned. "God dammit!"

A minute earlier I'd coaxed him to the window to see this strange animal move from the garden and scamper up the lone tree in our side-yard. After reminding me about the dangers of my imagination and the boy who cried wolf, he joined me there, said he couldn't see anything, turned to finish tying his bootlaces, fell.

Ted was gone, and Grandma, panicking over what to do, told me to stay with Grandpa while she drove the car down to Maple Lake to use a neighbor's telephone.

Half an hour later the ambulance came, backed up to the porch kitchen, and two men lifted Grandpa onto the stretcher, placing him in the back. One of the men, attempting to ease my fears, told me not to worry. He said that my grandfather was going to a hospital and would be back soon.

I believed, during those frightening moments, that I would not see him again, and I pleaded with my grandmother to call the men back. She explained that I would be able to see Grandpa as soon as he got fixed up and we could get into town.

Grandpa came home in early fall, took up life in his rocker, and spoke often to no one in particular.

"Get over here, you!" he ordered. "Tell that son-of-a-bitch I'm coming."

Grandma took me aside, told me that he was going blind and couldn't hear. I fed him scrambled eggs from a green plate each morning and held steady the saucer with his coffee before trudging off to school. Each afternoon I returned home hoping that he would somehow be better.

One night my grandmother stacked two cardboard boxes next to the bed where Grandpa lay breathing, deep. She draped a white cloth over the boxes and set out a cross with two candles in it. She lit the candles and told me that a priest was coming.

Grandpa was fighting for air it seemed, staring at nothing, a pale fleshy net between his white lips. That same thick smell of old sweat was present in the room, and had been for days.

It was dark when the fat priest came. He kissed his silk scarves, and performed secret rituals with water and a silver urn filled with smoke.

I wanted Ted to come see, witness the unusual spectacle, and I hurried into his part of the house to ask him.

"No, Yimmy," he answered quietly. "Don't see much in dos tings."

The priest called me into the bedroom, ordered me on my knees, then asked my grandmother why I didn't know the Sign of the Cross, jerking my little hand around my forehead and chest until I got it the way he wanted before reciting his hopeless chants. If the priest had invoked the name Roosevelt or Truman or Eisenhower or Oscar Biggs (a neighbor everyone talked about because of his size and weight) or the Lone Ranger and Tonto I might have understood, since those names were familiar. But praying long solemn oaths to what Grandpa and Uncle Marvin had always cursed, was confusing, and staring at flickering shadows dance across the smoky ceiling while praying long solemn oaths to those curses was even more confusing.

After the priest left, Grandma said I could crawl in bed with Grandpa. I slipped into the feather mattress beside him, listened to his slow rasp until I fell asleep. It wasn't Grandma who woke me, but aunts Noreen and Angelica. They directed me to my army cot, tucked me in, and told me I would sleep better there. Sometime later, as light shafts seeped through the curtains, there came an incredible wailing, and my grandmother came in, took me from the cot, hurried me behind the bedroom door, snuggled with me into our old coats and wept. "He's gone," she cried. "Grandpa's gone."

In the small graveyard my cousins and me, silly with cheer, scramble after smoking brass shells flung from volleys of rifle thunder. I pour the hot casing from one hand to the other before putting it safe into the same pocket where I keep my red-handled Lone Ranger jackknife.

After the burial, my aunts and uncles, my cousins, friends of the family, gathered in our yard at the creamery house. Cars are parked in the shallow ditch on the far end of the garden, and lined one after another on the garden's south edge along our driveway. There is a card table with a tray of cups and a large coffee pot set up outside our porch kitchen. There is another card table with a tray of glasses and a pitcher of red nectar. There are chocolate chip cookies and peanut butter cookies in a pan. There are bottles of beer in a wash tub filled with cold water from our well pump.

Those not speaking to one another stand separate each in their own group, talking of Indian summer, laughing, smoking, or doing nothing at all in particular. I have led those cousin friends nearest in size to my stagecoach in the creamery ruins. Six or seven or eight of us are up there riding furiously, and I hold the reins tight as we sweep around the garden and back through the yard, tilted dangerously one way then another with wild wheels spinning over rock and brick and earth and gravel. Another cousin takes the reins and another and another until each of us has had a turn, and then I lead them off the stagecoach down around Ted's garage where a corner opening between fence posts allows us entrance into the grassy banks overlooking the slough. We move in dancing leaps and happy twirls through thistles and burn weed and rotted tree limbs to the narrow path on the ridge where I speak almost without breath of what has come to pass most recently in my life.

It is here, I say most sincerely, that the Lone Ranger and Tonto ride up in late afternoons and meet me. It is here, on this very path, that we speak, I say, and see the hoof prints there and there and there. The Lone Ranger and Tonto appear the same as they look like on radio, I say, and it is here, on the spot we are now standing, that the Lone Ranger first lifted me for a saddle ride on Silver. My arms round his waist above his gun belt and my cheek against his shirt spine, and we take off on Silver full speed round the slough like you wouldn't believe and I mean lickity split. It is also here, I tell my cousins, that the Sioux ride up near nightfall, slide off their horses, and sneak up the hill behind Ted's garage to look at the garden where they once lived. They are savages, I say, and howl at the moon when they're sad and when they're mad one arrow through the heart is what you might get and you're dead.

My cousins, excited to be with me in this place on the ridge path, have agreed that I should be the chosen one to ask the Lone Ranger if he would please, please give each of us a silver bullet the next time he rides this way with Tonto, and they make me promise to watch out for the savage Sioux and, after I promise and say cross my heart and hope to die, we all seem happy and we run in a line back up the way we came and I'm first.

By sunset most of the friends and neighbors that knew my grandfather had gone, and my aunts and uncles, my cousins, old Ted, my grandmother and me have wandered into the garden. No one can say what led us there in this hour on the earth or what we are doing between the rows or what we should do or what we will do. But we are all together in the garden, and some are standing in one corner near the pumpkins, a few in another corner and some in the middle rows. Those of us so cleverly disguised as children are scattered here and there, some leaping over what's left of the carrot rows and others talking, looking, running, pleading for something or other, and we are all there when Aunt Noreen or Aunt Angelica or Aunt Digna – someone – mentions Regina and in the calm of the evening the word is clear.

This has happened before. Evening whispers outside the porch kitchen. Lowered voices at other family gatherings and in other gardens whenever I wandered near. And why is this? Why these mid-sentence pauses from my aunts as I rushed past, their words hushed, swallowed, gulped, eaten, spelled out, and locked behind a finger held to tight lips? And why a sudden enthusiasm from uncles sometimes forcing a brief but peculiar interest toward me, cryptic grins below large eyes that seemed brighter than the moment before, exaggerated delights masked by something with no name, and what is behind those unexplained glances of quiet sadness not easily disguised from children? And why, on this night under the first star over our garden, the day of Grandpa's funeral, the day when our good people gathered – brought the yard to spectacular life with genius cousins goofy with giggles, alive with thoughts of the Lone Ranger and Tonto and the Sioux who creep through darkness; oh why, on these generous days, potato salad and bean days, sweet nectar and beer and cookies days; why, when the grownups stood outside the porch kitchen from dusk into darkness and the moon above the yard light over the old ruins gave us kids extended play – safe from night ghost; why, when the adults moved from the garden, called us with cruel authority from our adventures dancing around the burning barrel, gathered each to their own family in whines of protest, ordered them to cars with me to stand and watch; why, as they counted their chattering little ones pleading always to stay a little longer; why, after they soothed regret, promised return, ordered a shush to silence – why, oh God why, oh why, oh why, I asked myself over and over and over, did they have to leave our yard again and again and again and again without once telling me who I was, and what was happening to my Mommy?

A pair of whistling swans, mated for life, has descended on Downey VA. The swans, rare in their grace and elegance and notorious for their disgust of ducks and geese, broke the water's calm and chased away the other foul in splashes and hisses until they were alone.

Patients inside 125-D have gathered not at the ward windows or the three-season porch to view the important new arrivals, but near the nurses' station where "lover tweet" the happy little canary, lies lifeless at the bottom of its golden cage.

Dorothy Gunderson and Velma Adams claim they witnessed Regina Van Amber reach in and strangle the helpless canary. "She did it," they say. "We saw her!"

William Williams, the black man Regina had cursed, and fought with more than once, comes to her defense and says the little bird died of old age and nothing else.

> *Physician Notes*
> "July 1 '53. Lobotomy Staff approved lobotomy. See staff chart. Operation will be scheduled after ward decorating completed."
> Taylor Scorba, MD

By late July, Morrison had become impatient. Regina's pre-lobotomy work-ups (EEG, skull X-ray and blood work) had revealed no abnormalities, anything that would prevent a "successful lobotomy". But Maxwell Sirca, Downey's chief administrator, had told the Lobotomy Staff that even though the vote was unanimous, he would like one more research study done on Regina. He pointed out that she had only been in full restraints for a total of six hours this year, and that was a significant change from the year before.

Morrison believed he knew the real reason behind Sirca's attempt to delay the "operation" and he didn't like it. Sirca was aware, like a lot of people around the country, that Lobotomy was fast losing the favor it once had with the nation's press. Relatives of alcoholic and schizophrenic patients were beginning to express serious doubts. Deaths due to brain hemorrhage were not uncommon. Post Lobotomy suicides were not uncommon. Walter Freeman, the medical celebrity who had introduced lobotomies into the United States, had turned into a kook crisscrossing the country with the words "Lobotomobile" painted on the sides of his van, telling audiences that he was a "headhunter". He'd had his picture taken while "lobotomizing" actress Frances Farmer in Western State Hospital near Fort Stellacombe, Washington. Freeman's supporters had even elected him president of the American Board of Psychiatry and Neurology.

It is hard to argue with titles and trophies. A few years earlier Freeman had traveled to Stockholm and presented the Portuguese Neurosurgeon, Egaz Moniz, with the Nobel Prize for Medicine. Moniz had drilled holes in patients' heads, poured alcohol on the frontal lobes to destroy them. Freeman was an admirer of Moniz and Morrison was an admirer of Freeman.

The psychiatric world, including the VA, had once again gone overseas (EST was introduced in Italy under Benito Mussolini) for the latest techniques in "treating" the mentally ill. In a very short time, without long term documentation or research, six countries had legitimized the process of changing human behavior by destroying the frontal lobes and, by 1950, over 30,000 human beings had been mutilated in the US and Canada alone, several more than once.

After Freeman returned to America, he happened to notice an ordinary ice pick in his kitchen drawer one day and, believing it had potential as a surgical tool, had it redesigned by a Chicago firm so it wouldn't break off inside patients' heads the way other surgical tools had. He began collecting royalties on his "invention". Within months following the ice pick's ominous redesign, he was putting on shows around the country, performing his lobotomy act in theaters, inducing electric shock or drugging and mutilating one patient after another before gasping crowds. Audience members often fainted during these lobotomies. Yet Freeman took each opportunity to discuss and promote his "Trans-Orbital" by proclaiming its benefits for those whom society could not control, avoiding the reality that most of his victims were women and children, or that the "operation" was irreversible, that people died from brain hemorrhage or that he was not a licensed neurosurgeon.

The VA continued to perform lobotomies. The second edition of the book *Psychosurgery* was on every psychiatrist's shelf by 1950, and in every medical school library. A lobotomy was cheap, quick and, according to Freeman, required only a pair of sunglasses to cover black eyes following the procedure.

"No worse than a visit to the dentist's office," Freeman had once said.

One month and three weeks after Regina's lobotomy had been approved by Morrison, Scorba and the Lobotomy Staff, the second research study Sirca had requested was completed, noting that Regina remained a "difficult patient with no plans for the future". The original decision to change Regina from someone who verbally and physically resisted to someone under complete ward control remained unchanged.

At the same time, far from North Chicago, an event was taking place that may or may not have had a direct connection to what had been planned for Regina in Downey. The world's top psychiatrists in Vienna gathered to hear the closing speech of a weeklong international conference on mental health. Professor Nikolai I. Oserazki told the world, and the *New York Times*, that lobotomies had been "banned" in the Soviet Union because they were found to be "cruel and inhumane" and "lacked foresight for advances and more therapeutic methods".

United States government officials who monitored the Soviet Union on a daily basis weren't surprised by Oserazki's statement, and even though many American psychiatrists in attendance agreed with the Russian's assessment, nobody who had an important desk in Washington paid much attention to the news. Three days after the story ran, however, those officials (along with almost everyone else of adult age in the US) came to attention, suddenly frightened by reports that inside the Soviet Union a massive hydrogen explosion had taken place, powerful enough to level any American city, and the second such explosion ever. The government had wrongly believed that the Russians were at least three years behind in their hydrogen bomb development, and US officials, not to be outdone in propaganda wars, began listening more intently to every word the Soviet Union said about anything, including lobotomies, piston engines, vodka and so on.

People were scared.

The word went out from the highest levels of government to all agencies, including the VA, to be sensitive to Cold War propaganda.

❖

Regina was in the Pack room on September 9, 1953. She had been in Pack for six hours. She was quiet under the wet sheet lumps when the nurse, following an unexpected call from Morrison, pushed aside some of the sheet humps, peeled part of the main body sheet off Regina's shoulder, then stuck her with a double dose of Sodium Amytal. She wasn't agitated. She wasn't squirming. She wasn't shouting "obscenities". She was dozing.

Morrison showed up in Hydro a little after 3:30 p.m. He wrote down the words "scheduled dental appointment" on her chart, and ordered the nurse to stick her with yet another double dose of Sodium Amytal. He checked Regina's pupils, made certain that she had no resistance, and with the wet sheet still wrapped tight around her body asked the nurse and two aides to lift her from the Pack bed to a wheelchair. Once she was in the wheelchair Morrison wrapped a loose sheet around her mid-section, tied it behind the high wooden frame, pushed her off down the hallway to the elevators and took her to his second floor office. The next notation of Regina being in a wheelchair wouldn't appear until 1979, twenty-six years later.

After securing Regina's head with a restraint belt affixed to the wheelchair's frame, Morrison set the brake on the wheelchair so it wouldn't move, and brought out his ice picks and a wooden mallet. He took one pointed steel in his right hand, pulled up Regina's left eye lid and tugged it away from the eyeball. He stuck the needle's point onto the section of bone called the "conjunctival sac" on her tear duct, careful not to touch the skin or eyelashes with the steel probe. He moved the point around until it settled against the sac, dropped slowly to one knee, aligned the shaft with the angle of her nose, exerted pressure and, with the mallet, the judgment of forever, struck the head with the sound of a dull snap, then pushed the point through her skull and into her brain. When he reached the five centimetre mark on the instrument he stopped, stood, and with his hand still on the pick's hammer, pulled the handle up toward him as far as it would go (stopped by the ridge of her eyebrow), guessing that the fibres at the base of her frontal lobes had been partially severed. He brought the pick back to its original position before driving it deeper to the seven centimetre mark. Then he moved the shaft about fifteen degrees downward toward her mouth, pushed it back to its original position, then pulled it about 30 degrees to the left and thirty degrees to the right. Morrison withdrew the steel spike by twisting it, at the same time placing pressure on the eyelid to prevent a burst of blood. He focused his attention on her right eye, and with the other instrument repeated the insanity.

The entire mutilation took less than fifteen minutes.

Morrison didn't concern himself with family consent or Walter Freeman's own warning that prefrontal lobotomies on extreme psychiatric cases were not recommended.

When Nurse Markam approached Regina's bunk to administer Serpasil medication later that afternoon she found her curled under her blankets, sobbing.

"Regina doesn't live here," Regina cried. "She's been murdered!"

I am sitting on a large rotten tree trunk above the path overlooking the slough. The Lone Ranger is nearby on his mighty horse, Silver, and Tonto is back and behind a little on Scout and both are looking not at me, but at something or someone in the distance near the rim of Maple lake.

There is always silence between us, only the sound of squeaking leather and horse snorts mixed with calls from the whippoorwill and the meadowlark and the redwing blackbird.

I am lucky to be near them in their time of danger. I am lucky to know they are here and I am here, safe, and when they ride, they ride swiftly, sometimes with me, sometimes not.

I try to explain to Grandma how much the Lone Ranger and Tonto really, really like me. I tell her both have taken a personal interest in my life and that everything will be all right. She says we might want to think about moving to town in a few months and I shouldn't be going into the woods or the slough alone. "You could be with a lot of other kids your age in town," and wouldn't that be nice?

At night she prays to Jesus and Mary, Mother of God, and I think about the Lone Ranger and Tonto and Grandpa and Regina.

One bright afternoon before the corn was fashioned into tepees that will dot the north cornfield like an entire Sioux village, I wandered after a pheasant that soon disappeared into the tall dry stalks. The sky was hopeless in a cornfield. I became lost and ran down a row that had no end then ran back to no end and my stomach hurt and I wanted to shout, scream for Grandma or Ted, but I couldn't. It wasn't the Lone Ranger or Tonto that saved me that day, but a woman who seemed perfectly at ease moving up the rows, smiling. I'd been warned about gypsies. She was dressed in a bright red pants suit, booted and tight to the skin. Her hair was the color of copper. Her eyes green and bright. She took my hand and led me to an opening in the back yard near the edge of the garden. If she spoke at all I don't remember what she might have said. It was one of those times when everything seemed very still and sound itself had no place to the ear.

Photograph

Less than two weeks after the unauthorized prefrontal lobotomy, Regina's brother, Edward, drove through the gates of Downey. His Brownie box camera was on the seat beside him next to an overnight case. After registering at the information and security building just inside the main gate, he found a parking place within sight of the pond and got out to the squawk of ducks and splashing water. The day was warm, a few clouds, with only a slight September breeze. Edward had driven from Montevideo, Minnesota, to spend a few days with his sister Angelica and her husband Lyle who had just moved from rural Minnesota to Racine, Wisconsin, an hour's drive north of Downey. Edward hadn't seen Regina since the time before she was taken from the old creamery house. The last letter she had written begging him to take her from the state hospital was still in his wallet, folded, hard as a coin.

He used the rear view mirror to straighten his tie, run a comb through his hair. He took the camera off the seat and got out. As he shut the car door, two nurses happened by on their way toward the gate. Edward wanted to make sure he was headed for the right building, excused himself, and asked the two where the female section was.

"We just came from there," one said. The other turned and pointed to the pond and the building not far from where they were standing. "All the female patients are at our Fall carnival over there."

Edward thanked them and moved from the parking lot to the sidewalk that followed the slope along the pond. Not far away there were large painted cutouts of cartoon animals braced with boards and bricks on the sloping lawn. Nearby, a small group of patients and aides were heaving horseshoes. One woman was cackling and the sound reminded him of a bantam rooster. Other patients were gathered around a bean bag toss. Edward was pleased that the weather was nice enough for the comfort of short sleeves and more pleased that his closest sister was participating in fun outdoor activities.

About halfway to the largest group gathered near the water's edge, two patients stood with their backs to him just off the sidewalk. He couldn't make out his sister in the distance yet and decided to move from the sidewalk, to cut across the grass to get closer to the main gathering.

"Hey, mister!" a female called. "Are you a doctor?"

He stopped and faced the heavy woman who was standing just off to his right with the other patient.

"No. I'm looking for my sister," he said. "Do you know Regina Van Amber?"

The woman grinned, her eyes sparkling with some instant knowledge before laying her hands on the broad shoulders of the patient next to her, spinning her toward Edward, and at the same time nudging the woman forward a little. "This here is your Regina," she said.

Edward stood helpless from the instinct to step back, call out his fear, stunned by mere sight of the woman's shocking presence. She was in cuff restraints, her hands positioned squarely behind her back, her elbows even. Her eyes were not visible, funneled above ravaged cheeks, a sad face puffed ill like the rest of her body, as if she had been recently dragged in death from the pond, propped upright, and put on display to rot in the sun. Here's what happens! Her face was swollen, punished, robbed of all dignity, all humanness; a sad, sick, horrible, tortured, primordial face, as if a gene from a Neanderthal had worked its way down several thousands of years from the last female, stopped with Regina, and stayed. There were scabies on her left shin below her knee, below her slip, exposed half an inch below the hemline of the thick hospital gown which had a huge flower embroidered for a pocket.

She stood adjacent to a tall cardboard cartoon bear who sported one suspender and trousers like Li'l Abner. The large woman next to Regina was more relaxed with natural eyes and arms folded, hinting at belligerence and at the same time presenting herself as being sisterly and protective toward the victim next to her. Regina's face was sorrowful, swollen and puffy, numb from the shock of daylight, numb from anything fresh and clean outside, numb from the secret ice pick. In her deepest darkness, Regina resembled someone who had lived years in a cave trying to focus now for the first time on life, trying without much success to get a view of this speechless disgust called living.

Edward clenched his jaw, moved closer, still stunned by the shocking image of this fleshy monster that had once been his sister.

"Regina? It's me. Edward. Your brother, Edward."

"Take our picture," the other woman demanded. "Go ahead. I'll stand right here next to your sister, doctor, and you take our picture. Are you the one married to a Jap woman from Cleveland?"

Edward didn't answer, didn't know what to do, what to say, except what he'd been repeating.

"It's me, Regina. It's Edward."

Regina said nothing.

"Take our picture," the woman was more forceful. "Hurry, before the German comes."

Edward retreated a few steps to honor the woman's request,

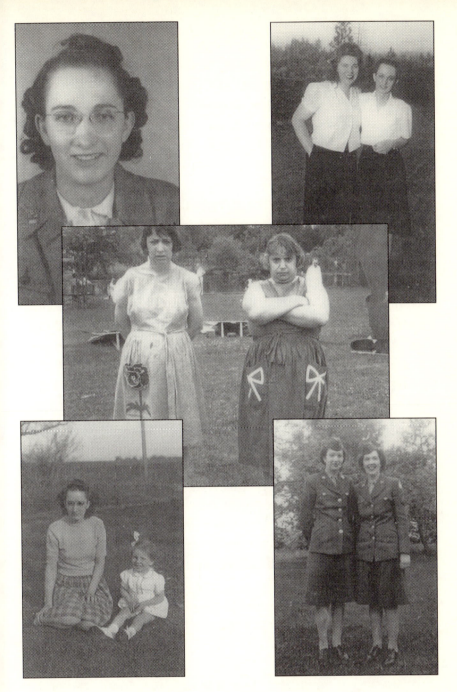

(Top left): A young Regina Van Amber before being hospitalised. (Clockwise): Regina with her friend; as a WAC in the military; with a niece and (middle photo) with another inmate of the VA hospital (left) when she had put on weight.

still not sure now how to act or what to do or what to say or what to think. He lifted the camera, held it steady while he cupped one hand over the viewer to block the sun, then peered down at the reverse image in the small glass magnifier. He snapped one frame, didn't really care whether the picture turned out or not, lowered the Brownie, and moved closer to his sister.

"Regina," he said. "It's me, Edward. Your brother, Edward."

"She don't remember you, doctor. And she don't like you either," the woman rambled. "You better leave now before we sink."

Edward called to his sister again, repeated his own name as if he was hearing it for the first time. And he called her name again this time with more emphasis, the same way someone calls a child out from under something. And he called his name again, and again, and hers again. But he couldn't take it, not five more seconds. And without words, without embrace, without a single touch, without looking back, without talking to anyone else, he retraced his steps to the car, tossed the camera on the seat, reached inside the glove box, took out a pint of whiskey, sunk low in the seat, and sucked down more than a few long swallows. When he felt he'd had just the right amount to drink, he swallowed one more.

A few minutes later, after he drove out of the main gate and turned west down the hill, he told himself there was no reason to return, no reason for hope, no reason for much of anything involving Regina. The vast swelling brilliance of Lake Michigan, in his line of sight for the first time, meant nothing.

Lipstick

During Christmas vacation, two months after Grandfather passed away, my grandmother told me she had made arrangements for the two of us to move into Alexandria, that it wasn't right to live with Ted anymore because Ted was a bachelor, and what would people think? I told her to marry Ted so we could stay. She laughed for the first time in a long time, said that was impossible, said living in town would be better for everyone. The decision was final, she said, reminding me that we had talked about this once before and that I had already said good-bye to my teacher, Hattie, and friends in the township school.

"You can finish the second grade in town," she said.

My teacher had told me that I would do well in the new town school, and that I was as smart as anyone my age. I was too fearful of the unknown to share her confidence, and could not see myself attending another school.

A Christmas storm delayed our move. The announcer on the Silvertone said the weather might be bad for days and I hoped it would be bad for weeks. Wind howled through the night bloating the wool blanket Grandma had tacked inside the porch kitchen door. Each morning we huddled close to the flames on the kerosene stove while Ted warmed himself near the wood burner in his part of the house.

The creamery table was under a dune of wind-driven snow. The well pump was almost covered to the pump shaft. The driveway had disappeared, no longer separate from the garden. There was no movement on Maple Lake Road. Massive icicles, pillared every few feet outside the porch kitchen windows, caged us, and the door was snowed shut.

The delay meant more time to talk my grandmother out of moving, list all the reasons why we must stay.

Once during the snowstorm, Ted brought out a fiddle and filled the small house with a snappy tune. I don't remember the song, but I danced near his stove hoping to somehow convince my grandmother that these were the best times.

After the road-grader cleared the snow and we shoveled out the driveway, Uncle Marvin came with his pick-up, helped load our boxes, our Sears Silvertone, our lamp, the cot, the featherbed, cords, the wringer-washer, our lives.

I was huddled on the far side of my uncle's old Ford when it came time to go. Ted called my name, and found me. I had knelt at the running board, buried my head on my arms and turned my back from the sad thought of seeing him for the last time.

"Go away, Ted."

"You're a good boy, Yimmy," he said. "I see you sometime when I go to town. Remember, Yimmy, I show you how to tie shoes."

The roof of my mouth felt hot and awful.

Old Ted was outside the porch kitchen as we left the yard, drove north past the mailbox. When I looked back again he was near the garden's edge where he could see us turn onto the road to go east. Grandma said she thought he was crying. I kept him in sight as long as I could, told myself that we would be back soon and talk to him, meet the Lone Ranger and Tonto on the path, and make sure to tell the savage Sioux they were welcome back in the garden anytime night or day, rain or shine.

❖

In Downey, that week, a student nurse found Regina hiding behind the latrine door. There was a large welt on her right cheek, and a couple of smaller bruises on her left arm. She was crying.

The four little white houses face a large dirt yard in the center of the block. The little houses look the same, sitting at a right angle from Fillmore Street, with short sidewalks, small square patches for front yards, and one small step.

We moved into the third house. 1213 1/2 Fillmore. People called them cabins, but they were more like roadside motel units that had been moved from some other place. The first two cabins stood separate. Our place was connected to the last cabin where a young married couple lived. The woman was pleasant to watch. She had long blond hair, blue eyes, and perfect teeth. We shared a laundry room with the couple, a wash-sink for soaking clothes and a frightening tin shower stall. Water shot out from the nozzle with enough sound and fury that I thought my skin would peel, and I'd go deaf. I didn't take many showers.

Two small windows looked out to the gravel cul de sac where dump trucks and bulldozers were parked. Each truck had large black letters on the doors that read: "We Move the Earth".

The landlord lived in the main house overlooking the street. The cabins, the house, a separate garage, trucks and bulldozers, the cul de sac – all of it was dwarfed on the east end of the yard by a high wall of honey-bricks, the back of a building large enough to cast long shadows in the morning. Grandma explained that the building belonged to the Coca-Cola Company.

The little cabin made me feel laughingly rich. The walls

were shiny, made of knotty pine. There was a solid door to the bathroom, hot and cold running water in a sink next to the toilet, a mirror that opened to white shelves (rusted in the corners), a toilet paper dispenser and four curious slots in a shiny metal piece above the sink. "We'll have to buy you a toothbrush," Grandma said.

The kitchenette had a gas stove, and we set our milk and butter in a small window. There was a space heater in the living room, and it meant no more wood or coal to lug, no poker to stick in the stove's belly.

In one corner, on a dark wood stand, was a telephone. It was solid and heavy like stone buffed to a dull black, brightened by a dial of numbers. The numbers, Grandma said, were our numbers exclusively.

All these marvelous things made me wish Ted were with us to share our fortune.

Six days after we settled into the small cabin Grandma drove me to Lincoln Elementary School, a new, one level structure on the west side of town. We checked in at the principal's office and, following a nervous delay of paperwork, the secretary escorted us to my second grade classroom in the building's south wing. The teacher introduced me to an entire room of second graders, walked me to a bright new desk, and explained how to elevate its top. After the agony of watching Grandma leave, the teacher announced that we would be attending a safety meeting in the lunchroom where each of us would receive fire hats. In the lunchroom, the man who came to talk with us and present us with our gifts was the same man who had come with the straitjacket draped over his shoulder, the man who had given me coconut candy, told me that my Regina would be home before I could say Jack Robinson.

Whether my blackout was caused by the actual sight of this

man I don't know, but I have no other memory of the second half of second grade or the entire third grade. My report cards have teachers' names, comments about shyness, not working up to my potential, and missing many days of school, yet my only memories of that time are those first minutes of second grade, the man in the lunchroom, and nothing else. The memory block would have served me a lot better, I think, had it lasted one more school year, extending past Miss Lillian Wein's fourth grade class. On the first day of school, Miss Wein asked each student to stand, say something about his or her family. I agonized over what to say, but when it was finally my turn she spoke for me. "Jimmy Van Amber lives with his grandmother."

Miss Wein was a double-chinned, bitchy perfectionist who reminded me of a giant hawk in red, jumbo glasses. She was a power pincher. She dug her nails into my ear and the nape-of-my-neck and my shoulder and my upper arm and my wrist. Her pinches made my eyes water. They hurt. She pulled my hair – jerks and tugs – and made me write: "I will not stare out the window" five hundred times every day after school for a week and "I will do my homework" a thousand times every day after school for another week.

She taught me how to loathe school, fear her red grade book, her hate book, her book of irreversible, red ink hells. She was the first person, other than Uncle Marvin, that I consciously feared. Weekday mornings were dread. Lining up in the hallways, kick-ball in the gym, and the triple click when I raised my desktop were all magnified with fears. I feared failure with the flute-a-phone, flash cards, spelling tests, grammar, recess and eating in the hot lunchroom where Eddie Martin said I was crazy for drinking my milk too fast. Grandma made me lunch for school after that, and I ate in the cold lunchroom, and I avoided any cafeteria for the rest of my school days.

REGINA'S RECORD

Miss Wein's classroom meant danger. I had trouble with arithmetic. I couldn't concentrate. I wasn't sure what she might do if she found out that I didn't yet know how to tell time. The fear of being held back became overwhelming at times. When I went to the bathroom, I stayed as long as possible. I faked stomach-aches and headaches, and prayed the school nurse would send me home with a diagnosis of something terminal, something so desperately wrong I would not have to return.

Sometimes, when I wasn't out in the hallway serving out some punishment, Miss Wein shamed me in front of my classmates. "What *is* wrong with you? Haven't you learned *anything*?"

The rest of my days in her class – time without end it seemed between the first buzzer and well beyond the last – Miss Wein made life in her room, under the disguise of elementary education, a childhood prison. I wasn't alone in the prison, of course, but had no way to articulate that to others who felt the same way.

When I opened my final report card, saw her signature allowing me to move onto the fifth grade, I believed, at least for a while, that she had made a mistake and the school would soon discover the error.

During that same time, Grandmother mentioned that Lillian Wein graduated high school the same year as Regina, but I had no understanding what that could have meant. In Mother's high school yearbook, Lillian Wein, future Teacher of America, was voted "Best Dressed Senior Female" and proud of it.

On ward 125 D, Regina was refusing to put on clothes. She told aides that if they were going to strip her in Pack anyway, she might as well not wear clothes. Her continued ability to fight with aides, and her verbal defenses on the ward, troubled Morrison and Scorba. It meant the Lobotomy, which literally was supposed to cut out hysterics and emotional outbursts, didn't take. But something else did.

On February 10, 1954, a nurse and three aides had come into the sleep area to wake her, tell her she had visitors waiting just outside the ward door. And for the first time the nurse wanted her to take a new pill, a tiny white tablet in a small paper cup. Regina slapped the cup off the tray, cursed the pill, and struggled to push back the aides. The fight continued from the bunk area into the hallway not far from where Uncle Marvin and Aunt Digna were standing, waiting, looking through the wire window.

"Your brother and sister-in-law are here to see you, Regina," the nurse tried to explain.

"I don't know what you're talking about," Regina shouted. "I don't have any relatives."

Marvin and Digna were bawling. They knew nothing about the lobotomy let alone any idea that her severed brain track was the reason for her memory loss.

A nurse tried to console the couple. "Perhaps you can visit another day when she is feeling better."

Digna explained the distance involved, that it might be some time before they were able to make the trip again.

"We'll take good care of her," the nurse said.

Regina was offered a second tablet later that day. She refused. She dumped a third offering on the floor and crushed it into the heel of her foot. There were sixteen more refusals. One nurse attempted to slip a tablet into her coffee. Regina saw her, and for ten days didn't drink coffee, demanding they not try to trick her again. Near the end of the month, nurses talked her into swallowing her first psychotropic pill, believing that the numbing effect of Thorazine (as it had for some few others on the ward) would somehow have a settling effect. It did not, but the staff wanted to believe that it had, and her restraint time over the next several months decreased to 36 hours.

Young Mr. Henry Aaron was playing baseball in Milwaukee.

The VA had no policy on the use of Wet Sheet Pack. There was one permanent Pack bed in the third floor Hydro room on 125 D, and my mother had been its regular, long-term occupant. By the end of 1955, she had spent 628 hours and thirty minutes wrapped in a wet sheet, stuffed into temporary submission and control.

Workers came onto the ward at year's end, removed the Pack bed, Hydro tubs and water tank. The sheets went down to the laundry and the wall hooks were unfastened and discarded.

Regina had been in Downey VA less than thirty-six months. 3,200 volts of electricity had stunned her body. She had been in full or partial restraints for 504 hours and thirty minutes, dropped into insulin induced coma 282 hours, had three "courses" of "Electro-Narcosis" (Shock and Insulin combined), suffered three "cataleptic" seizures, and 129 Grand Mal seizures. She became "assaultive" or "resistive" or "fighting" or "verbally abusive" or "fearful" on 542 occasions. She tried to escape twice, became the subject of two research studies, was attacked by other patients thirty-six times and fainted at least twice. She was exposed to tuberculosis, given 2,832 hypos of Sodium Amytal, underwent an unauthorized prefrontal lobotomy, and suffered countless bruises and abrasions. Countless. She fell on six occasions, and six times she was pushed to the floor.

The words *Sodium Amytal* were used most often in her progress reports. *Pack* or W*et Sheet Pack* or *Sedative Pack* were used almost as often, and the third most often used nota-

tion is *Lipstick*. "Lipstick is smeared today". "Lipstick has not been properly applied". "She is drawing lines on her legs with lipstick". "Messy lipstick on patient's chin". "Smudged lipstick" and several dozen other similar notations.
The word "screaming" appears 497 times.
Taylor Scorba and Manley Morrison left Downey VA near the close of 1955.
Christmas Eve she was on the bathroom floor behind the door, a place she often sought refuge. She had been in a scuffle with Lulu Martin, another patient, and had struck her forehead on the wall. The nurse reported swelling, but as "nothing serious" and did not call for the Officer of the Day. New Year's night she curled in her favorite chair near the radiators in the Day Room. She ran her fingers through her matted black hair, cursed "Mr. Lincoln", cursed the Japanese, talked about the importance of the flag, and how horrible it was to lose your child on the Lusitania (she'd seen a poster once with a woman holding her baby, descending below the water, with a caption that read: Loose lips sink ships). She rocked in place, watching, waiting, companionable with her demons before aides called for her to sleep, perhaps a chance to dream of lovely things in a garden somewhere safe beyond the beyond.

In our little kitchen in the Fillmore Street cabin we have green plates and blue plates and orange plates all with matching saucers. If anything breaks Grandma glues it back together. We eat Malt-O-Meal some mornings and oatmeal on other mornings and sometimes Grandma makes pancakes and speaks of the threshing crews that she used to feed when she was a girl. Sometimes we eat scrambled eggs. Sometimes, when I'm bored, we set up the card table and play Chinese checkers or seven-card rummy. She always wins. I ask her

REGINA'S RECORD

why she always wins and don't let me win. "If you win, you win," she says. "Why should I let you win? You shouldn't be a sore loser." Then for the umpteenth time she tells me the story of the man who felt sorry for himself because he had no shoes until he saw a man who had no feet.

I have learned to hate this story. It doesn't seem to have anything to do with Chinese checkers or seven-card rummy or anything else.

In spring she gets permission from the landlord to start a little garden beyond the last cabin near a tree. I know about gardens, she tells me.

Mary Jane Forbes

The word of Regina's memory loss and deterioration spread to each adult family member. Marvin and Digna told Grandma what had happened on their visit to the place, talked about what Edward had experienced a few months earlier and said they didn't know what to make of it. I overheard some of what had been said, and learned more later, but most of the communication about Mother naturally took place when I was at school.

"Regina didn't know who we were," Digna had said. "She's gotten a lot worse."

Grandma didn't understand this at all, she told me, and planned a trip to see for herself. "She would certainly know her own mother."

Grandma picked at her arm scabs whenever she spoke of Regina. There was almost always a spot of blood on her tissues.

I suspected any trouble with concentrating in school meant that I was becoming like Regina. My belief was based on the idea that Regina had lost her mind, had to be taken away, and anyone who has lost their mind, has lost memory and forgotten what it was like to be a kid.

To compensate, in case someone questioned my memory, I prepared myself the only way I knew how, and began a ritual of memorizing the total number of certain objects and where they were near the cabin. That way – if someone gave me a test – I could list one thing after another until they were satisfied that I wasn't *crazy*. Who *they* were, I wasn't sure. But there are six old truck tires leaning up against the rear of the Coke plant, I would say. There are eight pallets, oil cans in a big barrel, three oil drums, twenty-two pop bottle cases, fifty-five pop bottles with their necks broken, three batteries, a roll of wire, two metal signs with the words "Drink Coca Cola" in red on white. And while I resisted memorizing most everything in text books – I was baffled by much of it anyway, and it seemed uselessly boring – I told myself never to forget the stubby index finger on the school librarian's left hand, the missing little finger of classmate Darla Peterson's right hand, the kid's name (Darnel Baker) whose uncle's left eye was popped out by a hockey stick.

I told myself not to forget Mavis Molde (a second grader) who was run over by a drunk driver seconds after getting off her school bus. I memorized what Kay Warpy, a doctor's daughter, wore to class. If her father ever came to school and questioned my mind, I was prepared to rattle off what his daughter had worn, and he'd rightfully declare me mentally fit. He'd say, "Nothing wrong with this young man." Light brown corduroy dresses and a white blouse every Friday, I would say, and brown slacks with a red blouse under a blue pullover sweater on Mondays. Sometimes I couldn't keep up with the combinations, lost track, and thought about how I could divert my shortcomings to others. I would tell the doctor that Gordon Carlson put on earmuffs even when it was warm because he thought his ears stuck out too far and the muffs would help flatten them permanently to his head.

It was a lot of work.

That was the same time I ran into Ronnie Packer, a sixth grade bully who shouldered kids hard into wall lockers, then laughed. I saw the stunned glaze of submission in Ronnie's eyes when I told him that my mother was in a bughouse, that my father had just murdered four people on his way home from prison, that I had killed my grandfather, and that I lived alone in a fish house across the tracks. Ronnie Packer got his information while lying on the lavatory floor. My nose was an inch from Ronnie's nose. I was sitting on his chest. My hands were around his throat. His hands were around my wrists. We were sweating. Snot was running over his lips. He was pleading for mercy through those scared eyes about to burst into tears.

My worst fear was to be forced down on my back, pinned. Where this fear came from I didn't know and could not connect it to what happened to Mother in the yard. When Packer called me a retard, he used his fatty leverage and worked me down near the urinals. My fear was overwhelming. After a rolling scuffle, I somehow grunted my way on top, screamed the fake family history in his face, and told him to leave me alone. It worked. He didn't so much as toss an angry blink my way again. No one else did either. The word was out and it traveled. No other fights in that school or through junior high and high school. I didn't like fighting, anyway. Fighting made my mouth dry and my knees weak. But it also made the story I'd told Ronnie Packer too dangerous to own. The story needed control, a refinement of reality – the straightest, shortest line to the protection of pity. Memory was my security, but pity became my answer. Pity was justice and mercy combined. Pity was genius to me, a workable method of acrimonious posturing, and a reverse revenge.

Quite by accident, in Cliff's Little Store just across Broadway Street, I learned the importance of my story on adults. Mickey Ericksen, the blond clerk, was someone who seemed interested in the details of my young life. He was a stutterer, friendly, dense, asthmatic, with double thick glasses. When he asked about my parents and I told him whom I lived with and why, he appeared physically changed. He blew his nose. His brow furrowed with lines of dedicated interest. No mother. Mental hospital. Don't know father. Grandpa dead. "I live with my grandmother."

When the owner wasn't around, Mickey rewarded me with extra candy for my nickel, but the labour of listening to him work out his words made it more of a hassle than a coup.

My fifth grade teacher was a man. I wasn't sure what to make of him at first until it became obvious that his main subject – the thing he loved to talk about most – was baseball. Mr. Hawkins explained to our class that he was a baseball player for the local town team.

"I'm a catcher," he said. He had forearms like Popeye. He talked about baseball as if it was far more important than school. I dreamt of being his son. He would announce it in class.

"Jimmy is now my son," he would say. "He will be a baseball player too."

I didn't know much about baseball, didn't own my own glove yet, but in early fall that year he told us the exciting tale about the New York Yankees playing the Brooklyn Dodgers in the World Series. He spoke of these games in such a holy way that I no longer stared out the window wishing the school day was over. The blackboard became unimportant. Who cares about the clock? I felt rocketed into another dimension that required little work and no memorization. Sometimes, when his talks went on too long and I felt guilty, feared for him, I wondered if they were going to fire him for being a traitor to schoolwork.

For the first time since the one room school I felt safe in a classroom. In the spring we went outside to play kitten ball. I wasn't sure how to hold the bat, when to swing, where to run if I did hit the ball. The other kids laughed. My stomach hurt.

I would never be a baseball player.

Outside the classroom, there were always the questions. Almost every kid I met had questions. "Who is your Mom and Dad? How come you live with your grandmother? Why is your mother in a hospital. What kind of hospital?" There was no escape from the questions. What I thought the story needed were changes and additions to the story. Father killed by Germans during the war. A box of gold medals. Friend of Audie Murphy. Mother works as a nurse in a mental institution. Chicago. We see her when we can. She's very rich. She has a ranch and ponies. I live with my grandmother behind the Coca-Cola plant. We own it. Free soda whenever I want, everyday. (This story didn't last because it turned out that the parents of a younger classmate did own the local franchise and, once again, I was forced to shrink the story and revert to a line of pity).

What was troublesome was remembering which kid I had told what story to, and again (depending on who it was) plead my current state of aloneness, lowliness, and seek out a level of worth by being different, worse, unlucky, at the same time remain important and deserving like the Lone Ranger before Tonto found him lying on the canyon floor, shot, dying; Tarzan before Jane or Robinson Crusoe before Friday – anything close enough to be declared a lost orphan any moment.

The story, in many ways, became my perverse comfort. Who could not feel saddened by it? Who could not resist the desire to know more? The best and shortest version of the story, however, turned out to be the real one, stated as one quick fact after another before moving on to ride our bikes or play Davy Crockett, King of the Wild Frontier, or trading President cards.

REGINA'S RECORD

Sometimes, perhaps every two weeks or so, Grandma drove us to see Aunt Noreen and Uncle Frank on their farm. We always passed Old Ted's place but he was never outside and we never stopped. The garden was covered with weeds, no longer neat with those long rows my grandmother had so labored to make perfect.

That same summer, in Noreen's garden (a place almost surrounded by woods), Noreen said she saw something that disturbed her and she screamed and the family said she had to be taken to a mental hospital like Regina. No one said what it was that frightened her, but I knew it wasn't the Sioux. I'd asked Aunt Noreen once if she'd ever found arrowheads, mashers, and scrapers – anything like that. She told me that the only thing she found once was the skull of a cat.

Grandma told me that she was worried sick about Noreen. "And all those little kids," she said. The family of six children my age and younger was split up. Two went with neighbors. The oldest two stayed on the farm with their father, Frank, and two were sent to an orphanage in St. Cloud, sixty miles east. We drove there once. The two boys, Greg and David, were running toward us down a long dark hallway when we first saw them. Three nuns in their black habits were behind telling them to slow down. Both my little cousins had puckered up and were sobbing, asking about their mother, wanting, begging to come home with us. Grandma wept for an hour on the trip back. "This world," she said, "is a bad place."

Aunt Noreen came home in the Fall and her children joined her and Uncle Frank. A farm neighbor had tended the garden and, when we went there for a visit, my six cousins and I ran between the rows, plucked out the fattest carrots and ate them until we were stuffed.

Whatever Noreen had seen and heard in the garden was

gone and no one dared say anything about it again, least of all us kids.

In town, there was this one person near my age that I met early on who had her own sad tale and, for the first time, when our stories met in a shared experience, there was no chance to become anything other than delighted equals and like me she knew nothing about baseball.

We saw Mary Jane Forbes before she ever saw us. It was our first morning in the little cabin.

The crow of a rooster moved us to the bedroom window. Grandma cleared the frost with the edge of a comb, looked out to someone's back yard. I'd heard roosters crowing in the country, but the expression on Grandma's face and the surprise in her voice suggested that this was a rare event in town, rare enough to wonder out loud where exactly this rooster was and whom he belonged to.

Through the frosted pane the wind kicked up snow swirls to an outlined blur of a figure in a plaid scarf, someone bundled portly from the cold – a ghostly image of speed running from the back porch of a large house to a small shed.

"It's a girl!" Grandma exclaimed. "She's gone to feed her rooster."

Who this mystery girl was and how she came to have a rooster we didn't know but, when the weather was nice enough to play outside, I burned around the first cabin near the street to this smiling girl running toward me across her front yard. I stood dumb as a rope while she grinned a head above me, and said: "I know your name. Your name is Jimmy and you live with your grandmother, and you go to Lincoln School. I've seen you there."

Meeting Mary Jane Forbes was an event not without consequences, yet her timing in my life was perfect. Spring to early summer, with the sweet smell of lilacs in her backyard near her garden, Mary Jane became my explainer, pony tail swinger in a white blouse and orange peddle-pushers, kid-good in bobby-socks; the girl next door, hula-hoop talent and, far more importantly, the first person who, like me, had no parents, no brothers or sisters; a person who raised the least of my defenses; someone, my grandmother said, who had a story far too dangerous, too tragic, too horrible to ever want to repeat to her face – something about a car crash on a slippery road at night. I'd never heard of anyone dying in a car crash.

Childhood misery seeks justice through friendship. Our friendship grew. Each day when the weather was good we met in her back yard near the edge of her aunt's garden where she had set up a tent. We read Alcott's *Little Women* aloud as we obligated ourselves to sip invisible tea.

Mary Jane was exciting. Her knowledge and humor impressed me. There was no sidewalk on our block, so we played across the street on the steps of a small white church on the corner. Mary Jane speculated that people who came to this church rolled on the floor and spoke strange oaths while the other parishioners clapped and wagged their tongues and shouted to heaven. She said that the minister actually approved this rolling around even though all the women and girls were ordered to wear dresses. She said they were very strange.

Mary Jane showed me what a television looked like through a neighbor's picture window one Saturday morning in the rain. She told me which boys threw rocks. She taught me how to ride a bicycle, jump rope, twirl a hula hoop, play jacks and hopscotch, and pointed out which sidewalk cracks should not be stepped on under any circumstances. She took me to my first movie, and pointed out that Ma Kettle (Marjorie Main) looked exactly like my grandmother. It was true. After the movie show we ran home and quizzed my grandmother about it. Grandma laughed, but the idea seemed to appeal to her, and the next time a Ma and Pa Kettle film came to the Andria Theater she took me and marveled at the female character.

Sometimes, during hot summer nights, while cricket chirps rose to meet the dark, I overheard Mary Jane's uncle shouting furious demands. His voice was angry and cruel – a wicked man, I thought – someone to be feared when he drank, and to avoid when he didn't. I used the comfort of my pillow to block out the bark of his rage and hoped Mary Jane was doing the same.

One morning we heard a nervous rapping. Mary Jane's presence surprised us because it was the first time any neighborhood kid had knocked on our door. And there was something decidedly different about her appearance. She was pale. Her lower lip was puckered. There was a look of hurt in her eyes. She was out of breath. She begged me to come outside and talk.

I wondered what I'd done wrong.

"People who run the town said I can't keep Crow," she cried. "Mean people."

Watching his glorious strut in the wired coop that day, we discussed Crow's fate, how we could teach him not to crow, wrap his beak with electrical tape, hide him out until he learned to control himself.

"Don't be foolish," Grandma said after I told her of our plans. "That's what roosters do. He'll be better off on a farm."

Mary Jane and I were not able to reason this out. People had all sorts of animals in town, she said. The very hatchery where Crow came from as a chick was inside the city limits. And there was a man in the town who kept snapping turtles, goats, garden snakes, worms, geese, dogs that didn't stop barking. How does he get away with it?

Mary Jane's uncle took Crow away, and sunrise was no

longer broken by the rooster's noble announcement. "I'm never eating chicken again," she swore. But Mary Jane did eat chicken, and after she ate chicken we met in the gravel yard and spoke of her suffering in low cautious tones, defeated by nameless forces more powerful than hope or love.

That summer I first discovered the horrors of organized youth baseball, joined a little league team that played behind the American Legion two days a week and asked Grandma if she would buy me a glove. She said we could not afford one, and then brought out this weird fat thing from a box under the bed. "Regina used this sometimes in the yard," she said. It was stuffy, thick and ugly and old with stubby fingers and a pocket that bulged with strands of stuffing loose near the palm. "Authentic Ty Cobb" was still visible in the center. I brought it to the games, prayed that no one would hit a ball to me, prayed my name wouldn't be called to bat, prayed that no one would notice the old glove.

Playing baseball meant suffering that summer, and brought about fears I never thought could be overcome. Besides possible embarrassment in missing a ball hit to me deep in the outfield, it became apparent that during my plate appearances something happened that did not happen with the other kids. Parents who cheered for their offspring or for some neighbor kid they knew, were suddenly silent when I approached the plate. I didn't dare turn around to see what had happened, what this silence was about: why everyone unexpectedly stopped talking, but I suspected something was terribly wrong with the way I looked, the way I held the bat. I suspected the small crowd had noticed the old glove hidden under the bench and couldn't believe anyone would be that stupid to bring it to a game. I checked my zipper to see if my barn door was open. It was like standing naked with boils covering my entire body not sure how they got there. I began to avoid the games, and decided to forget about baseball and its heartache and especially after this one kid told me that my very absence had cost my team the championship because the final game had to be forfeited. I vowed not only to never set foot on a baseball field again but instead to dedicate my life to becoming a hood and talk about boners, smoke Camel cigarettes, walk around swinging a bicycle chain, and grow my hair long enough to comb into a magnificent duck-tail.

Mary Jane said I was just being mean to myself and told me to stop it. She took me into her garden and we sat between the rows of sweet corn and she said that I needed to stay closer to her because she was not a boy and not mean and who cares about hoods.

Grandma and I rode the Great Northern when we went to see Regina in Downey for the first time. It was an exciting journey with a friendly conductor and his silver hand-punch snapping tiny holes through tickets. Riding the train was magic, an adventure hard to sleep through. Everyone appeared pleased to be in motion, and we were in motion with them. We ate hard-boiled eggs, bananas, egg-salad sandwiches, and potato chips Grandma had packed for the trip. She said eating in the dining car was too expensive. Traveling by train, waiting in vast depots, listening to the staccato list of towns and cites over the loudspeaker, greeted by smiling red caps Grandma was always suspicious of because she said all they wanted was a tip, seeing friendly conductors – all of it made me feel important and part of the excitement in the world.

Aunt Angelica and Uncle Lyle picked us up at the train station in the great city of Milwaukee before they drove us to their home in Racine. Our second or third day there, my uncle drove us to North Chicago. The day was hot. Uncle Lyle and

REGINA'S RECORD

I sat on a bench not far from the pond while Grandma and Angelica went into one of the buildings.

I imagined Mother looking at me from one of the tall windows, pointing out how much I had grown, what a good boy I was. I wondered when she would come out or when they would call me to go in. My heart beat fast thinking about it.

"They don't allow children," Aunt Angelica said after they exited the building.

"Regina doesn't remember me," Grandma said in a stunned voice. "I think she would have remembered her own mother."

I felt hurt by the exclusion. Like someone had jabbed me in the stomach. Grandma sobbed all the way back to Racine.

> *"Patient's mother from Minnesota visited today. Ward aides complain they can't get within ten feet of Regina."*
>
> Maxine Lambert, LPN

"Forty-Seven Days in August"

By January 1, 1957, almost five years from the date of her admission, Regina had been in full or partial restraints for a total of 752 hours. Counting Wet Sheet Pack and restraint times, she had spent 1,371 hours in some form of physical restriction.

The latest medications after Thorazine – Stelazine, Pacatal, Compazine, Reserpine, Sparine, and Trilafon – were supposed to allow her the same freedom others had experienced, but in Regina's case VA doctors decided to experiment by a concoction of *polypharmacy* (mixing antipsychotic drugs). Since there was no research or information on what effect these medications had on someone who'd undergone a prefrontal lobotomy, the VA apparently guessed at what the dosages might do without consideration of side-effects.

On February 1, 1957, an hour after Regina refused to participate in Music Therapy, six aides and two nurses took her from the Day Room into the sleep area on 125 D, forced her on her back, notched a thick leather belt snug around her waist, put restraints on both wrists, hooked the restraints to metal eyelets on each side of the belt, put her in "anklet" restraints, wrapped another belt around the entire bed frame and over her stomach, notched it, threw a blanket on her, and left.

That was Friday.

Eighteen hours in full restraint.

The next day, twenty-one hours "without relief" and the

REGINA'S RECORD

next, Sunday, three hours without relief, and on Monday six more cruel hours.

There was an eight-day "break" while the medications were mixed and the doses elevated. In the first criminal stretch, from the twelfth to the twenty-fourth, Regina was in full restraints for an average of eighteen hours a day.

She was squirming, struggling, attempting to twist free, calling out, begging, cursing, screaming, defecating, tossing in dreams, urinating, vomiting – held at the mercy of her keepers for no less than six hours, then eight, ten, twelve continuous hours, fifteen continuous hours, eighteen, twenty, twenty-one, twenty-three hours at a time.

Four times a day during these brutal periods, nurses lifted her head, saw to it that she swallowed the drugs, and a trickle of water. Dosages were increased when it was apparent there was no change. By the end of April the mixed antipsychotics were maxed-out at their highest recommended levels and, by the end of August, my poor mother, helpless and confused, had spent 789 hours and forty-five minutes in restraints with four psychotropic medications fighting against each other in her body.

789 hours and forty-five minutes.

> *"Beneficiary Van Amber is calling out this p.m. She said there cannot be forty-seven days in August."*

Mary Jane told me that a new kid was moving into the corner house next to her place. "A boy my age," she said. We were standing near her garden when she told me this. She sounded sad. "His parents are rich," she said. "I suppose you'll want to meet him."

A day or two later, after the moving van pulled up to the blue, ranch-style house on the corner and workers began bringing out furniture and boxes of all shapes and sizes. Mary Jane and I watched from the steps of the little church across the street. Mary Jane was right. The kid was rich and I did want to meet him.

The Pit

Peter Wilson wore Hush Puppies, knew Latin, was an altar boy, could recite the *Gettysburg Address*, and *The Midnight Ride of Paul Revere*. His parents drove a white Thunderbird and his house had an outside antenna for their color TV. His mother, a quiet pleasant woman, had a Veg-O-Matic with extra cones, and there were cloth place mats on their kitchen table and carpet in the living room and carpet in the basement and carpet in their spare room and carpet in a basement bar. Everything seemed to have a place, and everything that was in place I thought I had been born without. Electric Football, Monopoly, Clue. He had a ping-pong table, a basketball hoop and net above the garage door and a brick patio with a picnic table and grill. He had his own bedroom, a record player, a closet full of clothes, and a battery operated robot named Robbie who said, "I am Robbie Robot, me-chan-ical man. Drive me and turn me wherever you can."

I always felt a little cheap in Peter's house, took my shoes off in the entryway and always checked my socks to see if any holes exposed my skin.

Peter told me one day after we first met that he was from Wisconsin, a town called Waupun where there was a hospital for the criminally insane. The patients there, he said, would wring your neck for no reason.

I didn't tell him about Regina right away. Didn't want to ruin my chances with him.

Each Sunday Grandma and I attended Mass in St. Mary's at the north end of town. She had told me that the church was made of Kasota stone from a quarry not far from where she grew up. "The Philadelphia library is made of Kasota stone," she said.

Whenever Peter served Mass he seemed to know exactly what to say and what to do and when to do it. His confidence about life was appealing.

After church, Grandma and I usually stopped at Osterberg's Cafe on Broadway Street and ate orange doughnuts. Once we ran into old Ted walking to his car. He said he'd just come from the Red Owl store where he'd picked up his monthly supply of peanut butter, jelly and bread. He seemed pleased to see me, asked how I was getting along, said I was growing like a weed, asked how I liked town. "How do you like town, Yimmy?"

Ted usually ran out of words after a sentence or two because whenever we did see him on Broadway Street (about twice a year) the conversations were brief. "Place is still the same. Car runs good. Weather is good. Getting along good. Oh yah. Yah oh yah."

Grandma told me that, since Ted had lived alone most of his life, she suspected that whenever he came to town he strolled a few blocks hoping to see people he knew and I was one of them. "Too shy to ever come for a visit though," she said.

More than once, after getting back from Peter's house, my grandmother made comments about spending too much time there and that my attitude always changed. "What about Mary Jane?" she asked. "She is still your friend, isn't she?"

"You don't understand," I replied.

"Just remember," she said, "you can't keep up with the Jones'."

Peter had introduced me to Elvis songs. He played them over and over on his record player until we had the words memorized.

During spring when the weather was warm and the scent of lilacs was once again everywhere, Peter, myself, Jerry Pranskevich and Jerry England (two other neighborhood kids) hung out at a square cement window pit on the north side of the Coca Cola plant. Peter sometimes dropped into the pit, and started singing, *Are you lonesome tonight? Do you miss me tonight? Are you sor-ry we drifted a-part?* Peter's voice was deep and strong just like Elvis. Peter was good.

The edge of the pit rose a foot above the level of the grass. Dropping into the pit was no problem. Peter was the best at climbing out because of his height advantage, but the challenge, for the rest of us, was not to work our way back up red-faced and breathing hard. The two Jerrys and I had to make a standing leap from the bottom, catch the high ledge with both arms, then shimmy up the rest of the way.

Peter was the judge of who accomplished the feat with the least labor. "Your face will give you away," he said in a light tone.

We spent most warm days sitting on the edge of the pit. Traffic on Broadway tripled during summer, and our position at the pit gave us the best view to look for out-of-state license plates heading for the lakes north of town.

There was a nickel Coke machine inside the plant and we drained bottle after bottle, never quite satisfied from thirst, checking each bottle's bottom to see who came up with the bottle farthest from Alexandria, Minnesota.

Mary Jane knew of the Coke machine; she would come by

sometimes to get a Squirt or Cream Soda and never said much, except hi.

Peter taught us how to play chess in his dad's basement bar, and he never lost and the three of us suspected that he was withholding certain information about moves. One night when Peter was upstairs and his parents were gone, Jerry Pranskevich and I slipped a small bottle from the rows of large ones behind the bar, snuck out back of the house, sat in the bushes, said, "Let's get drunk," and took a drink. I went first. It didn't come out very fast, but what did was bitter, burned my tongue, my throat. "Jesus," I gagged. Jerry took the bottle, tipped it, and shook it into his mouth. "Kee-rist," he spat. We rushed under the nearest streetlight to see the label, make sure we didn't taste that brand again.

"Worcestershire Sauce," we read in slow unison.

It was the only thing I stole from Peter's house, and the guilt was so overwhelming that the next time I was there, I put it back.

These were the days when we often spoke of where the first nuclear bombs would fall when the Russians attacked us. The four of us agreed that it would be Washington DC, far enough away not to matter much. Peter got a hold of the book, *Peyton Place*, and we took turns reading the sentence about sex. "Anyone got a boner yet?" Peter laughed.

One day Jerry England got a baseball glove from his older brother who was stationed in Japan. The glove's webbing was shaped like Florida and it didn't seem possible that anyone could ever miss a grounder. The glove's leather had a light tint of yellow and green. Jerry let me try it on and it had the feel of another hand over mine.

During one afternoon at the pit, when a local football hero who'd played at the university drove by in his convertible, Peter called him a homo. The big man heard it, stopped his car in the middle of the street, leaped out, came up the lawn like a mad bull, and asked the four of us who it was that called him a name. Peter confessed, the man slapped him, and everything we'd gained in group power and fun that summer vanished. Peter ran home, and the rest of us were speechless, stunned with the new knowledge that the single utterance of a single word could bring about such violence.

> "While undressing the above name beneficiary who was in bed restraint, she was noted to have many bruises over entire body, notably on both shoulders, back & left hip as well as both arms and legs. Bruises were in various stages of discoloration, some appearing very old, others quite recent. When asked about bruises would only say 'I was born with them'".

Kathryn Manning had worked at Downey for five years. Early in 1958, she had put in a transfer request to work on 125 D, was granted the request, moved over from another building, and began a review of ward procedure and patients' files. She had a good sense of humor, liked her job, and felt she could contribute her skills effectively with female patients. Her husband worked in nearby Waukeegan and they lived not far from the hospital.

By mid summer she was appointed head nurse.

One new building (where the pond is) and two new additions had been under contract for construction in spring. Manning insisted that her closed ward patients be given more time off the ward not only to watch the building that was underway, but to participate in other outdoor activities like playing catch, extended walks around the grounds, shopping trips and maybe activities outside the hospital. Manning met with initial resistance from the administration regarding the latter. They voiced concerned about distribution of patient funds, elopement risks and problems of under staffing, but eventually her suggestions were granted. At around 12:30 p.m. on a Friday in the second week of July, 1958, after seven years of being in a locked ward inside the grounds of two institutions, Regina boarded a blue bus with three nurses, four aides, ten open ward females, and the six other patients of 125 D. They followed another busload of male patients from the wards, headed out the main gate, and turned south.

The OD that day had told Nurse Manning that Regina could have two dollars. The RN gave her a small coin purse and Regina folded the two bills and tucked them inside. It was the first and only time she would have money. Then the nurse suggested Regina put on a dress to look nice – something about seeing families with children, something about a great speaker, loud, would announce who they were and many people would see them. Regina wasn't sure what it all meant and she became fearful, but other patients were talking in excited tones about the glory of it, and things suddenly seemed possible, interesting, and maybe even fun. She decided not to resist.

On the route, she saw neighborhoods and houses and cars and sidewalks and garden plots. She saw women pushing baby carriages. A tricycle tipped to one side. A dog on a yard lease, barking. Some man in a suit. Two girls jumping rope, laughing. There were beautiful boulevard trees and neat lawns and front porches with wooden swings and when the bus stopped at a rail crossing for the passing rush of a thunderous train she saw more people going places.

Everyone on the bus seemed happy as if this was the only direction home or the best route to heaven, breathless and complete and filled with hope beyond measure. Even the agony of time began to right itself until someone said they might be late and being late was almost a sin and at least a crime. She didn't want them to be late. Not now. Not with great expectations. And when aides spoke of a certain man as if he were a young god she wondered who he was, until they spoke of another and another and she wondered who they were. They spoke of this man – these men – as if they knew each so well, everyone was family and holy, and right to be alive on this good earth. "Del" she heard, and Al and Ernie and Eddie and Lou – and Joe, twice. And they spoke of song and food. And the bus stopped and moved and stopped again and everyone filed out, moving in a line through gates where smiling men stood thanking each person for coming. "Programs," someone hollered. "Get your Cub programs here."

Rise above these earthly cares. Cast your eyes on this!

And they stayed in a line, walking finally through a short tunnel into brilliance so close you could almost reach out and touch the magnified greens and browns decorated with flour lines, pure and perfect. "Cold beer here." The place rose up, swelling around her like a large toy baseball park some neighbor children had erected in one day. Without warning, there came a great roar as they were shown to their seats along the right field corner where a ball had just hit and bounced back onto the field.

"There's Ernie Banks," someone said.

There's Del Crandall, Billy Bruton, Al Dark, Felix Mantilla, Joe Torre.

"There's Eddie Mathews," someone shouted. "He's good!"

Lou Burdette, Warren Spahn, Joe Adcock, Jimmy Goryl, Moe Drabowsky, Tony Taylor.

These great chants were rising and falling and rising again. Some booed. There were hoots and hollers and oohs and ahhs. There was laughter. The laughter sounded like music made by elves. Someone said it was the bottom of the second now and the Braves were coming out.

Regina watched them explode out of the dugout in a tight group before they moved with grace and speed each to their own place. The colored man who ran near and stopped and turned was holding his glove over his heart. How fragile is the heart? How near we linger near the gods who watch over us, smiling.

"Please welcome our veterans today from Downey VA hospital in North Chicago," the announcer said.

Applause rumbled again loud before it fell. Some stood longer than others, clapping.

"Hank!" somebody shouted. "Over here!"

The Black man with a clear strong face, handsome and quiet and dignified, caught the last rifled practice toss from Billy Bruton in the center, then, in almost the same motion, spun to his left and lobbed the ball in a long gentle arch toward his team's dugout. "Hank!" someone shouted again. He turned his head slightly and fixed his gaze on the nearby seats. His lazy eyes, large and serene and unblinking, surveyed the nurses and aides in their whites, noticed the others in the group who were waving toward him. "Hey Henry," someone hollered. "Cubs are gonna win today, Henry." He touched the red bill of his blue cap, grinned, nodded at the group, moved the glove from his chest, laid a soft fist with a twist into it once, then again, and once more, faced home plate, bent slightly and kept bending until his hands were riding on his knees just as Burdette kicked and delivered. He did not look their way again.

Regina had two beers and a hot dog with relish. For two and one half glorious hours in Wrigley Field, she was no different than any free and happy human being anywhere on earth.

The newspaper said the Braves were shaky that day. Lou Burdette was relieved in the fourth inning, and it appeared the

Cubs were going to win until Eddie Mathews smacked an inside fastball high into the right field seats a few innings before Del Crandall drove in Jimmy Logan with a clairvoyant single in the bottom of the eighth and that was it.

As the bus left Wrigley Field around 4:30 p.m., on the way back from the game, I was headed out the door toward the old hotel annex a couple of blocks from where we lived. Some Cuban ball players had come for a three game series during our town's summer centennial celebration, and they were practicing hook slides on the lawn next to the annex house. Dave "Baby" Cortez was on their transistor radio with The Happy Organ, and I was desperate for a way to find revenge for what had been a horrible summer.

Satchel Paige and the Cuban All-Stars

Grandma was frustrated by the little garden on Fillmore Street. She said she was getting too old to keep up with it, and it was a bad plot anyway, mostly gravel and globs of oil the landlord had dumped there. She said her gardening days were probably over and she mentioned finding a little apartment on the north end of town near the baseball park. The announcement that we were moving brought about fear and worry. I hated the idea of leaving my friends, but she reminded me that I was spending a great deal of time in that park anyway and wouldn't it be better if we lived close by, and nine blocks from Peter and the two Jerry's weren't all that far.

The little apartment is on the lower level of a narrow white house overlooking the baseball park. It has a refrigerator with an ice tray, cramped toilet with a tin shower stall where grandma stacks boxes, a mechanic's sink with two spigots, and a gas stove. The room extends from the kitchen area separated by a pale green divider with an eight-inch space to the ceiling. Grandma makes one half into her bedroom, and I put my stuff on the other half.

We had use of a refrigerator for the first time, made ourselves ice water, and talked about how food would keep longer.

I had been sleeping with my grandmother up until that time, probably woke with a hard-on pressed against her back one morning, and she wanted me out. I took up my side of the divided room on a sofa, put the Silvertone on a box at the head of the sofa, plugged it in, and instead of falling asleep to the music, heard every sound, every creak, every thump in that place as if it had been the original home to Poe's *The Tell-Tale Heart*.

The narrow house had four apartments. A ministerial assistant and his pregnant wife lived in the back apartment upstairs. Jim Ross, a pitcher for the town's baseball team, and his wife Lois, lived above us and the landlord, a woman who spent most of her time in California, kept her furniture in the back apartment.

I didn't like the place. The short musty hallway leading into our apartment was dark and gave me the creeps.

An Easter card from Downey, that Spring, arrived three months late, but it gave Grandma more hope in her voice than I had ever remembered hearing. I had been out playing whiffle ball with new friends who lived across from the park, hanging a four-foot curve into the wind, laughing at the ease of play. When I got home, Grandma showed me the card, pointed to the signature. "It's her," she said. "Don't you think?"

"So what," I answered. "What does it mean? Nothing."

I looked at the handwriting again. "Happy Easter," it read. "Come see me sometime. Love, Regina."

"It's not her," I said. "If that's her then how come she don't remember me? Huh? Someone else wrote that."

Grandma rummaged through her boxes, came out with postcards, compared the handwriting.

"I think it's her," she said again.

"I'm telling you it's not her," I shouted. "Don't be stupid!"

I grabbed the Silvertone and threw it cord and all against

the refrigerator. It ricocheted off the door and fell crashing on the floor.

My grandmother was horrified.

What I didn't tell her, and couldn't, was that I was more interested in knowing about my father not Regina. I had been watching friends' fathers, watching fathers in the movies, fathers who came to baseball games and I'd been dreaming about how one day mine would walk into my life, come into my school, impress everyone I knew.

I was secretly sick of being embarrassed when Grandma showed up for school conferences in her old gray coat, lumbering down hallways in a loud bulky dress with her slip showing and balls of tissues stuffed under her nylons in big brown lumps up and down her legs. She was seventy-three years old, knew nothing about baseball, girls, or fathers (or so I thought).

"I don't want to hear about Regina," I said. "Nothing."

The young minister had heard my temper tantrum, waited for the right opening, and a few days later talked Grandma into taking me on an overnight trip to northern Wisconsin. His wife was staying home, he said, and he promised we would be back the next day after he saw his parents.

On the trip he spoke of little else except Jesus and sin, and at one point on a big hill somewhere in northern Minnesota, he pulled the car over and ordered me to drive. I was more than surprised. I had never driven, had no idea how to do it, and told him so, but he insisted, threatening me by saying we weren't going anywhere until I drove his car. Once we started down the hill with my hands tight and clammy on the steering wheel, he extended his left leg, put his shoe on the top of my shoe, pushed the gas pedal to the floor, and asked me what I thought about Jesus now. I was terrified. There were oncoming cars and I thought we would hit them head on. He kept the high speed (how fast I have no idea) and repeated the same question, shouting in my ear: "What about Jesus now? What about Jesus now?"

How far we traveled with me behind the wheel I don't remember, but when we arrived at his parents' home in Wisconsin, and, after they showed me to a basement bedroom for the night, I overheard the young minister tell his parents that my mother was in a mental hospital possessed by demons, my father was probably in prison somewhere, my grandmother was too old to handle a juvenile delinquent like me and, when we got back, he was going to recommend that I be sent to a boys' home.

The city limits of Alexandria never looked better. My first question to Grandma, of course, was whether she would ever consider sending me to a boys' home. She asked where on earth I got that idea. I made up some story, and told her to forget it.

The minister's assistant and his wife moved out of their apartment a few weeks later. I didn't speak to either one of them again, and their decision to leave may have been based on the number of flat tires they'd been having when their car was parked in back. I didn't think much about their Jesus either.

Two weeks later (and whether this originated with the young minister I have no way of knowing) the local Elks club decided to round up all the young boys in town who didn't have fathers. The plan was to send us to a two week camp a hundred miles north near Brainerd, Minnesota. Grandma talked me into it, said it would be good to get with other boys like me and she promised that it was no boys' home, just a fun camp-out. "Besides," she said, "you'll get to see Paul Bunyan and Babe the Blue Ox." We never did.

"In an attempt to talk with Miss Van Amber about outside world, she stated, 'I've heard all this before. Leave me alone.'"

"For no apparent reason, patient Van Amber was slapped by patient Bernice Hoyle after breakfast this a.m. Assault form filed. No apparent injury."

"Miss Van Amber seems to be off balance most of time. Check meds."

Grandma drove me to the bus for my trip to camp. I recognized two or three of the boys, had seen them around town, but didn't know them well. Most had come from broken homes or their fathers were in prison. But it didn't take long to realize that this was no ordinary summer camping adventure. The first night there all the counselors got drunk and a fist fight broke out near our barracks. I felt completely alone and helpless. There were constant threats either by the staff or other kids. One older kid named Lowell established his power quickly and began naming everyone. A boy with an irregular shaped skull was called "Football". My name was "Flunky". Everyone had a name forced on them and Lowell said that if we didn't use the new names he would break arms: "Shit-head" "Dork-Brain" "Hair-lip" "Pussy-Face" "Homo" "Mongoloid" "Mommy's Boy". I thought Lowell might kill me. His eyes were like black ice. I prayed for mercy and protection every night, had a horrible time walking into the main cafeteria for meals and thought about throwing myself into the nearby lake.

REGINA'S RECORD

The head counselor, Butch Armine, said he'd been a Marine. After morning PT, Butch ordered everyone to board the buses and we headed into Brainerd where we visited the local jail. "Stay away from the cell bars," the jailer warned. "These men could be dangerous and might break your neck if you get too close." The counselor told us that we if didn't shape up we could end up here like these "tattooed losers". The next day or the next he invited a highway patrol officer to demonstrate what happens to criminals. The officer brought out a Thompson sub-machine gun and unloaded the entire clip into a grove of nearby trees. "That's what happens to bad guys," the officer said. "Don't ever get smart with the police."

Lowell jacked off in the shower each morning and ordered us to watch. I didn't have pubic hair yet and most of the other boys didn't either, but Lowell, maybe two years older, was sprouting a red bush and what appeared to be a full size penis. He told us that when he got home he was going to store his jazz in a milk bottle, set it in the refrigerator for girls who came over, then offer them a drink of "really good milk".

> "Miss Van Amber went bowling with group today. Took ball and rushed down lane before aides stopped her. Does this patient wear glasses?"

> "Miss Van Amber was assaulted on the ward this am. For no apparent reason, Patient Ginger McClarren struck Miss Van Amber on back of head and neck with a board game. No apparent injury."

"This SN asked Miss Van Amber if she knew how to play a tune on the piano. She got up from her chair, sat on the bench and played a simple tune. Then she used many vulgar terms at me and walked away at a rapid pace. As she neared the nurses' station she stopped and looked back at me and smiled. Then she did some dance steps, made an unkind gesture at me, and went into the bathroom and shouted continually the words, 'Why don't they leave me alone'. This went on for two or three minutes before she came back out and said in a very loud voice, 'I don't dance for just any worms.'"

The name Flunky followed me home and hung on for about two weeks until I got a cracked bat from one of the local baseball players after a night game. I toted the thirty-four ounce Louisville Slugger on my right shoulder wherever I went in the neighborhood. The name Flunky stopped because I was sure no one would dare lip off to someone carrying a baseball bat. But a week later, the day Mother had been to Wrigley Field, and the same day I first asked the Cuban players if I could be their batboy, I heard another name in reference to me. I had this vague idea that what they had said was cruel, but I wasn't sure how cruel until the great Satchel Paige came to pitch.

"This patient has been to Occupational Therapy 572 times and has made little progress!"

Norma Baker
Occupational Therapist

REGINA'S RECORD

❖

My idea of being batboy for the Cubans was an act of revenge against the Runestone Clippers baseball team for rejecting me as their batboy, and instead bestowing this important position on another boy. I suspected that this act of injustice toward me was a result of my fatherless life and, indeed, the other boy not only had a father, but one who at one time had played professional baseball.

I'd heard that Leroy "Satchel" Paige was the greatest pitcher of all time, had a fastball that hitters could not see, and would destroy his opponents with his arsenal of pitches. When he came onto the field that summer night, and the crowd of three thousand rose to their feet, my heart sank. He was old.

He called me over to put on his spikes. I felt important. He was wearing a Cleveland Indians uniform. He appeared as some ancient warrior, tall and thin and dignified, with long arm and hands that held a baseball is if it meant nothing. He pitched three innings and each pitch was a little more than a lob. I was too young to understand that the pitches were ceremonial, and Satchel Paige had come as a past legend, ineffective to the events I wanted to happen.

The Runstone Clippers beat the Cubans and Satchel Paige that night, and when I was exiting the ball park a couple of kids called me a "nigger lover".

I wore that harsh label with a kind of confused pride that summer, unsure about what it meant in its totality.

The end of my time in Central Junior High School had not gone well. I suspect it was due to my protection as a smart mouth, little irreverent remarks in class about this or that which most often put me in the hallway or the principal's office. Sometimes there was violence involved. In shop class,

Mr. Larsen, during a speech he was giving on the first day of school, overheard a remark I'd made to another kid, rushed to where I was sitting, kicked the folding chair out from under me, picked me up off the hardwood floor by the back of my jeans and shirt, and flung me across the room like a sack of potatoes. Other kids met similar fates, driven into wall lockers by an irate teacher who'd gone berserk over some comment. And while I never saw a student physically assault a teacher, there were plenty of times male teachers grabbed certain boys by their throats or shirt collars or put them in head locks or twisted arms behind backs before shoving kids out into the hallway. I met most of my friends in hallways.

I missed a lot of school, made dozens of seemingly plausible excuses and felt great relief when Grandma let me sleep until noon and hang around listening to the radio the rest of the day. Those days I did go, fearful of the stack of make-up slips in the principal's office, I sometimes avoided the first bell and the rest of the day's classes by hiding in the fire tunnels that ran under the building. Grandma always fixed sandwiches so I had enough to eat when I went to school, and once I was down in the tunnels there was enough light from wall vents to read *Classic Comic* books. And there were love notes and poems from the Forties and Fifties candled on the ceiling and Lucky Strike cigarette butts snuffed out everywhere. I tried to imagine what some of the people looked like by what they wrote and what circumstances brought them to the tunnels.

"Miss Van Amber is behind the bathroom door curled on the floor again this a.m."

"Miss Van Amber is talking loudly to 'Mr.

REGINA'S RECORD

> Lincoln' again this a.m. Check meds."

> "Miss Van Amber sometimes looks at a magazine, but her attention span seems short as she gets up, often walks away, then comes back."

Downey VA sent another single page medical permission form to my grandmother. It was the same dangerous form the VA had sent in the early Fifties. Grandma worried, took it to an attorney. He read it, crossed out any reference to "removal of tissues" and Psychosurgery, and made her a copy. But her effort meant little. That same week my aunt Angelica traveled from Racine along with Joyce, her daughter-in-law, and went to visit Regina on the ward. Angelica had been there before, of course, many times. Regina didn't remember her sister, of course, and the visit didn't last long. As they were leaving, a man approached, introduced himself as Dr. Merit. He asked Angelica if she would be willing to help out and sign a form so they could "do some dental work on Regina". Angelica signed and dated the form, Joyce witnessed it, and they left.

The form Grandma sent back to the VA by registered mail (she kept the copy) was missing from Regina's 31 year stack of final records that arrived in 1994, but the same form that my aunt had signed and dated on the ward, witnessed by her daughter-in-law, was included in the stack.

I had met Dick Richard in the hallway outside of English class and we became friends. He had suffered polio in his right arm and always wore a blue sling where he kept our cigarettes. He had an older brother who drank beer. One night my friend showed up at my place with his transistor and a six-pack of malt liquor. We walked a few blocks to a hill overlooking Lake Winona, took up a spot on the warm grass, used his "church key" and started on the beer. The moon was up. The night was calm, and the water was smooth. Somewhere between the first and second beer Roger Miller came on Dick's transistor singing his latest hit song.

"Turn that up," I said.

I had been waiting for a way to feel perfect about my life and the voids that seemed insurmountable and overwhelming. Suddenly it didn't matter. Nothing mattered. I was perfect. Everything was perfect. The simple answer had enlightened me three gulps into the second beer. "I'm going to do this again," I thought. And the night was better than good. The pleasing dark filled with a silly insignificance, swelled inside me with enormous excitement, a lightness rising from my chest, weights lifting, guilt gone. With my new freedom came a sudden, immense, ever-expanding joy over the discovery of a universal truth only I, and I alone, could fully understand. Goodness and love dwell in malt liquor. My inner world was singing high praise to the gods of alcohol.

"Whoop, whoop, whoop, whoop – chug-a-lug, chug-a-lug."

It was 1961 and Regina had lived on the third floor of old Building 100 for ten years, but the construction on Building 131 in the center of Downey was now complete and staff escorted female patients off 125 D for the last time. The group walked the short distance to the new building, moved through a hallway, rode the elevator to the fourth floor female section, and took up residence there.

"Miss Van Amber seemed to be in reality

> because she saw some workmen on the roof and stated, 'They're up quite a ways. I don't like heights myself. Do you think they get scared up so high like that?'"

"Yimmy!"

I had come up the basement steps from Harold's Pool Hall, a downtown tavern that catered to kids fifteen and older. The jukebox below was blaring a Beatles song. My friend, Dick, nudged me. "I think that old guy behind us knows you," he said.

It was Ted. He was standing sideways, holding a grocery sack, and shaking himself the way he always did. I hadn't seen him for a couple of years.

"Yimmy! You're getting tall," he said.

We shook hands. He asked about Grandma. "She's okay," I said. "Still getting around." I mentioned that she had sold the old car a few years back, didn't drive now. He seemed interested. It used to be his car.

There wasn't much else to say. He said that his health was pretty good. He asked about high school. "Getting through," I said.

After we parted, I told Dick that I knew what was in the grocery sack. "Peanut butter, jelly, and a loaf of bread," I said. "That's what he eats. That's all he ever eats."

"Weird," Dick said.

Harold Barsness, the deputy who took my mother to the State Hospital, was the county sheriff, and had been for eleven years. Whenever I saw the sheriff around town, I looked the other way, pretended I hadn't seen him, slipped into a doorway out of sight. His oldest kid, Tom, was in the same grade in high school. I managed to avoid contact with Tom, feared he might mention my name to his father and there would be talk.

Judge Baderlund lived three houses down the hill from our apartment in a stucco cottage across the street from the baseball park. Grandma didn't say much about him. I made no connection between the stout little man and Regina until later but, at the time, I didn't understand his peculiar interest in me – the strange comments, odd questions.

He walked past our place on his way to and from the courthouse every workday. Whenever I was outside sitting on the steps or in the side yard taking practice swings with my Louisville Slugger, he stopped, smiled, and greeted me.

"Are we thinking good thoughts about the nice day? Are we thinking about our future? Are we satisfied with school? How are we doing? Aren't we fortunate to live in such a wonderful town? Good big seeds make good little seeds. A chip doesn't fall far from the block. Are we getting along with Grandmother? Are we having positive thoughts this day?"

Every few months, Art Kolar, the local veterans' service officer in charge of parenting Mother's disability pension, and the man designated by the VA to act as her legal guardian, stopped by the apartment. He told Grandma there was money enough for me to attend college. Her funds had added up over the years, he said. Grandma never knew the actual dollar amount, and believed Kolar was honest with his management of the money. But there was no mystery to the concern in her voice.

We lived off Grandma's social security and a small pension she received as the widow of a Spanish American War veteran. We ate fried potatoes, corn and chicken, fried potatoes, peas and liver, fried potatoes, beans and hamburger, fried potatoes, carrots and ham. We ate egg salad sandwiches, fried egg sandwiches, fried potatoes, fried eggs sunny side-up, and toast. Once a month she baked bread, and a perfect lemon meringue pie with an extra crust sprinkled with sugar and cinnamon. Once a week we each ate a golf ball size roll of fresh raw hamburger with a pinch of salt. We ate tomato soup and chicken noodle soup. Once in a great while we ate rice. And one time we made pizza from a box, and it tasted exotic.

We never went hungry.

During a fresh winter dumping, my last year in high school, I was picked up by police for throwing snowballs. Three other guys and me had been lobbing soft missiles through a blind alley, had the bad luck of hitting a squad car. I was caught, taken to the police station, grilled about who my accomplices were.

"I was alone," I repeated.

"You don't have four arms, boy," one cop said.

"It'll go easier on you if you tell us," another said. "Who were you with? We want to know. Give us the names. How long do you want to sit here? We've got all night. We want the names, and we want them now, or you're not leaving until we get them."

They finally gave up after a couple of hours, wrote me a ticket and let me loose.

I appeared with Grandma in Baderlund's court a few days later. She mentioned being in that same room with Regina. Baderlund read the charge, asked for my friends' names again, warned me that we could have killed someone, repeated his demands for the names, and when I refused, he entered a guilty plea before sentencing me to sixty days probation.

My baseball coach, Charlie Basch, called Baderlund to

protest the penalty, but the judge refused to reverse his decision, said my lack of cooperation with police was a serious matter. The following week I jogged to the courthouse to meet with the probation officer. The officer looked at my file, shook his head, said he had better things to do, told me to behave myself, and said that he didn't want to see me again. As I was leaving he called me back, said there was one punishment he was going to enforce, told me to take a minute on my way out to read the names of World War II veterans on the bronze plaques near the entrance.

Mother's name was there. I'd seen it before, wondered what his request meant, looked at the names of my aunt and uncle, and left.

That night I met friends behind Harold's Pool Hall. We sat in a car, guzzled a few warm beers, acted goofy and enlightened, ran down the back steps of Harold's, ate Slim Jim's and Polish sausage, dropped money in the juke box, cranked it. Tommy Roe. Beatles. Jerry and the Pacemakers. Roy Orbison. The Rolling fuckin' Stones. The Searchers. Dusty Springfield. Frank Ifield. I liked Frank Ifield. Frank Ifield sings: *"I remember you, you're the one who made my dreams come true, a few kisses ago."*

Around midnight, eight or ten of us left Harold's and took the fire escape up to the dime store's roof, clapped fresh snow into ice balls, waited for a black and white to cruise by and, when one did, we pelted it, I mean drilled that car so full of sound it must have seemed like war.

We came down off that roof like lemmings, split up, ran ten directions back to Harold's place, came like rolling thunder down his steps, begged him to lock his doors, and he did. And he dimmed the lights, and the cops came by, pounded on the door just as a Leslie Gore record screeched to a stop. When the police left, Harold, who did not like cops and proved it on a regular basis, served up free glasses of 3.2 beer to everyone

except a kid named Ezekiel who was fourteen.
 I liked Harold. We all liked Harold.

I didn't speak to Judge Baderlund again, turned away, crossed to the opposite side of the street, looked down.

I wore my black and red leather jacket until July, played American Legion baseball, hit a home run in Fargo, hit one not far from the state hospital in Fergus Falls, hung out at Harold's joint until he decided to close, kept the cracked Silvertone on at all times, fell asleep to Dick Biondi on WLS in Chicago, won five dollars from St. Mary's Catholic Church for second place in a writing contest about Jesus, didn't give my grandmother anymore shit about anything, graduated with a D average, got drunk with friends camping north of town by a lake one night and woke in a cornfield groggy, bewildered, and naked.

In Downey, Manning requested a beauty parlor be set up where the old Hydro room had been. Shampoo basins, hair dryers, and mirrors were installed. Regina refused to enter fearing what might happen, that five or six aides would soon leap at her, strip her, wrap her tight like a mummy but, eventually, the student nurses coaxed her in. Instead of her usual chopped hair done most times in the past with force, she began to look like a human being, and, as one nurse wrote into the records, "smiled for the first time since the baseball game".
 Manning brought up other issues and insisted that full restraints be used during extreme periods of agitation only, and that at least one staff person stay with the patient at all times during any restraint period.

By the end of 1958, Regina had not been in restraints once.

What Manning could not change, however, were doctors' orders or the whim of some VA bureaucrat. The concoction of pills continued. Even those "special" days the VA Central Office in Washington specifically deemed their nationwide "Drug Holiday" where no pills whatsoever were to be distributed, Regina, at least, was the exception. She was swallowing an average of twelve psychotropic pills a day, every day.

Manning left 125 D, taking time off to have her baby. By the end of 1961, Regina was held in restraints again for 218 hours and thirty minutes and her demons were still coming, some human, most not.

The Everly Brothers are on the Silvertone. Rock 'n' roll is making me a better person. The Crests. Chuck Berry. Jimmy Dean. Miss Tony Fischer singing The Big Hurt. Dion and the Belmonts – oh wa oh, oh wa oh.

Tennie Stowe is an angel in art class. One kid told me that she was flat, but a nice person. Another told me that she belonged to a weird religious sect that didn't dance. But in the hallways and during class our eyes met with smiles and something inside me melted and something else made me feel light and pleasantly goofy. I tried to think of how Hank Aaron would approach her, ask her for a date, and find out if she did dance. I practiced a few times, of course, until one day during an art project I went to her, spoke living words to her – surprised they came from my tongue. "Would you go to the school dance with me?"

She said, "Yes."

I walked to her house. Music lyrics hot in my thoughts. *Raindrops, so many raindrops . . . falling from my eye, eye . .*

REGINA'S RECORD

She met me at her door, smiled. I walked her to the dance without the presence of gravity. We held hands in the dark gym while the music played. "Is it all right if we dance," I finally asked. "Yes," she said. "Of course." My fears were relieved. My stomach felt normal. We moved with ease to The Fleetwoods, *Come Softly To Me*. My right hand was on the small of her back, her soft sweater fabric made by an approving angel. I felt strong and gentle and decent and undeserving and rotten and stupid and clean and dumb as a rope.

Grandma continued to make comments about Regina but they seemed farther and farther apart. Most were in the form of questions. But she did always mention Regina's name when she sent greeting cards to Downey, sometimes wondered if she got them. One night after she went to bed she quietly repeated what she'd said a few months earlier. "I don't really think Regina could ever live on the outside again, Jimmy."

"Yeah," I said. "I know. So what? You've said that before."

Grandma sniffles and the click of her rosary beads sound like little teeth chattering in the quiet dark.

Whenever she mentions Regina to me now, the back of my neck stirs.

There is no record of anything about Regina inside Downey VA for fifty-three continuous days in 1960. No medication charts, weight charts, music therapy notations, occupational therapy records, no physical therapy notes, no doctors orders, progress notes, physical examination files, nothing.

The last notation in a progress report is dated July 15, 1960 reads: "*Agitated on ward this a.m. Check meds.*"

❖

The next notation of anything appears fifty-three days later on September 7, 1960 and reads:

> "*Beneficiary was coming out of the chow hall and slumped to the floor. She was pale and her pulse was thready. She stated, 'Isn't this the desert?'*"

My mother was supposed to be in Downey VA hospital in North Chicago, supposed to be on the closed ward, supposed to be there with other patients. But it goes this way. Each day, sometimes several times a day, for over thirty years, nurses, doctors, aides, and student nurses write something down about Regina, her meds, her remarks, her misery, her appointments, her refusals, and more. Yet, right in the middle of those years, fifty-three days are missing, blank, gone. And no one, not one VA official has explained what happened to those missing records except to say that "they just stopped writing it down".

Man On His Knees

It is Saturday evening, October 2, 1964, warm. Around five minutes to eight, on the fourth floor inside Building 131, nurse Kathryn Manning and two aides escorted the women out of C ward, down the elevator, then through the main hallway which angles off toward the movie theater.

Once inside, aides took seats behind the females on the right about half way down while Manning remained near the double doors, then took an aisle seat near the back. That way she could watch the film, and keep an eye on anyone who got up – needed to use the bathroom.

The theater lights dimmed to dark, a shaft of light burst under the ceiling flush and wide to the screen, and newsreel footage began to the sound of trumpets. A cartoon followed the newsreel, and by the time the main feature started, Manning had settled comfortably in her seat.

About fifteen minutes after eight o'clock, one of the double doors over Manning's left shoulder opened enough to allow in a slash of light before the shadow of a man slipped through. The man stood perfectly still for a moment, not looking at the screen, instead covering his face with both hands as he waited for his eyes to adjust to the darkness.

Manning saw who it was – recognized Robert Clayton – an open ward patient scheduled for release in a week. Clayton, a thirty-year-old vet who had suffered shell shock in Korea, slowly began working his way down the aisle, hunched, looking anxiously to his left and right.

"Robert!" Manning whispered aloud. "Who are you looking for?"

Clayton stopped, turned to the voice, made out Manning, smiled and retraced his steps to where she was sitting.

"Looking for you," he said, then knelt to one knee. "There's this young guy in the lobby. I ran into him back by the elevators."

"A young man? Who?"

"Didn't catch his name. Here to see his mother, he said."

"His mother? Who?"

"Regina Vamberg – something like that."

"Regina what?" Manning leaned closer. "Not Regina Van Amber?"

"Yeah, that's the name."

Mann relaxed in her seat, chuckling. "You're pulling my leg again, Robert. I know your game."

"I'm not," Clayton insisted. "He's here – in the lobby. I told him that you were the night nurse in charge, and that all the female patients were at the movie with you."

Manning rose from her seat. "Robert, I know you. And–."

"Hey!" Clayton's voice rose above a whisper. "Don't believe me? Go out there. See for yourself. It's the truth. He said that a patient named Regina Van Amber was his mother, and he hadn't seen her since he was little."

Manning was standing. "Are you sure he said Regina? It can't be. Regina doesn't have any children."

"Don't tell me. Tell him."

"You're coming with me." Manning took Clayton's arm. "If this is a joke tell me now, Robert."

The two came out through the double doors into the dim lobby. Manning saw a black haired young man standing near a wall near the entrance. Manning, still clinging to Clayton's arm, moved closer, then stopped, standing still almost as if an intuitive thought had warned her not to advance.

"Robert here says you are here to see Regina Van Amber," she said in a firm voice before advancing a few more steps, craning her neck forward. "Is this true?"

"Yes," he answered.

"How on earth do you know Regina Van Amber?"

"Regina's my mother."

Manning opened her mouth and held it for a moment.

"Are you – do you have identification, young man?"

"I have a student ID card," he said. "University of Minnesota."

"I don't believe this," she said offhandedly, then tossed a suspicious glance at Clayton who was beaming. "I cannot believe this. Robert here is always kidding around and–."

He handed her the plastic card and she bent toward the best light, then studied his picture like someone looking for indications of a forgery, stared at his ID a long time, it seemed, then looked directly into his face, examined his features as if she were searching for minute details on an old map, noticed the unmistakable piercing green-grey eyes.

"Good god, young man!" She pressed her chest with one hand, then reached out and touched my arm with the other. "I owe you an apology. I had no idea Regina had a son. And I've known your mother for years. I've been one of her nurses – years."

"Is she here?"

"Here?" Manning appeared confused, as if she had lost track of where she was standing. "She didn't come to the movie tonight. She's back on the ward. We can go there now and see her if you like."

We started back through the main hallway.

"Robert mentioned that you haven't seen your mother since you were little. Is that right?"

"I was five or six I think, over twelve years ago"

Manning started to say something, then stopped, and faced

me again. "Are you sure you want to see your mother?"

"Yes," I said. "I'll see her."

Is this the way I walked before? I didn't come through this way? I couldn't have come this way. There were people. Toothless men pinching butts from the ashtrays, laughing at something flying circles around their eyes. Where did they go? This can't be right. The hallway was much brighter, much longer, and we're at the elevators where I met the Korean vet, asked him where the women's ward was.

Are you certain you want to see your mother?

"Yes," I said, wondering why she had repeated herself. "I'm sure."

"Beg your pardon," she asked. "Are you all right?"

"Yeah, I'm okay. I brought some gifts. Is that okay?"

Are you sure you want to see your mother?

"She's on the fourth floor. There is a visiting room just outside the ward. I'll take you there. Do you want me to dress her up?"

"No, no. That's okay. I'll see her, you know how she is. How is she?"

"Good days and bad," she answered.

Are you sure you want to do this? The question, uninvited, was darting around in my head.

"Oh, okay."

A scream behind the ward door startled me. I pretended not to hear. We moved through a short hallway into the small visiting room. The nurse was saying something, smiling, saying something else. Her lips were moving.

The door shuts. I sit and look around the room. I stand and look around the room. I move to the window overlooking the parking lot where I came in. I'm not sure about this, maybe shouldn't have come here. I take out the gifts from my school bag, then place them on the white coffee table, positioning them a safe distance from the edge so they won't fall. One round cigarette lighter. Why did they make it round, anyway? Two packs of Winston cigarettes. I didn't know what kind you liked. Do you like candy? I've got candy, all kinds of candy. I've always liked candy. This box has a second layer underneath the white paper. Well, you would know that. Yes, I like baseball too. Grandma doesn't know much about baseball. Oh, she's doing fine. Still gets around good. Ah, ah, ah – I started college now. Don't know what to do, really. I mean my major. General education classes now. Any ideas?

I rearrange the box of candy, the cigarette lighter, the two packs of Winston. I'll sit here. She can sit across from me. I'll stand when she comes in. Maybe I should stand now. Maybe I should get a drink of water, clear my throat. Maybe I should wait and see what happens. I should maybe explain who I am. I'm James, I'll say. No, I'm Jimmy. I forgot to bring pictures. Well, Grandma has sent pictures. Do they let you –? do you watch TV? What's taking so long? Who was screaming? I've heard that scream. They're drugging her up. I should have listened to the nurse. What did she say?

Wait? Did she say, "Wait"?

I'll bring your mother here?

My mouth is dry.

Something is bad.

This room is small. The nurse locked the door, or does the door lock automatically? Someone is unlocking another door. I should have come in daylight. Time goes by so slowly. That can't be her yet.

"Hi, I'm–." "This is your son, Regina. I'll leave you two alone, alone – *alone, alone*. I'll be back in a while..." *before you can say Jack Robinson.*

"Take your time. Go ahead sit now, Regina. Don't you ever look nice. Don't you think she looks nice?"

"Yes. You look really nice. You didn't have to dress up." The nurse left. "I'm James. Jimmy. I'm your son, James."

"I don't have a son."

I don't have a son. I don't have a son. I've never had a son. You are not my son. You have never been my son.

Her fingers are dark brown. Cigarette smoke. How could she hold her fingers in such a way the smoke coats them brown? "I brought you cigarettes." She is sitting on the edge of her chair. Why is she sitting that way? Her hair is nice. "Your hair looks nice." Black like mine. "Black like mine."

I don't have son. I don't have a son. You are not my son. Who are you? Why have you come here? This is not a good place for you. Who do you think you might be?

Don't you remember me?

"I'm James. Do you remember me?"

"No, I don't remember you."

"You remember Grandma?"

"Grandma? No I don't remember her."

"Do they treat you okay in here?"

"Who are you?"

"I'm James. Your son."

"I don't have a son."

"I go to college."

"Are you a priest?"

"No. No, I'm not a priest."

"Why aren't you a priest?"

"I don't know. Do you think I should become a priest."

"No."

"I have this candy I brought. For you. And this cigarette lighter. It's round."

"Yes, it's round. I want to go now."

"Well, couldn't you stay a little longer? I mean, well, the nurse isn't back yet. Wouldn't you like to stay, please?"

"No. You should leave here. I want to go."

Her face is like mine. We look alike. She is whimpering, standing now, moving to the door. Oh jeez, I'm sorry. Don't cry. Please don't.

"Could we talk again sometime?" I ask.

She has on a dark blue dress with white collar. She is wearing nylons, and black shoes with straps. There is a small scab on one knee.

The nurse.

"Are you two having a nice visit?"

"Yes," I say, "but she wants to leave now."

"Okay, we can do that. Should I take her gifts?"

"Yes. Here. Take them."

"Don't you want to say good-bye to your son?"

"Good-bye."

I am facing the window, but there is nothing to see. The nurse has come back. She has moved behind me, close, her hand on my shoulder. "I know," she said. "I know."

Kathryn Manning had signed her name several hundred times noting Regina's weight, blood pressure, type and dosage of medication given, but she made only one narrative entry.

> "Visited by 18 year old son this p.m. for approximately 10 minutes. Was not aware Regina had a son. She did not seem to know who he was. She did allow him to kiss her on cheek."
>
> Kathryn Mann, RN

I have walked from Building 131 into the night, crossed the dimly lighted parking lot toward the main gate, wiping tears on my jacket sleeves, walking not wanting to look back, walking thinking about Regina's eyes, how her unblinking stare seemed to penetrate walls, and me, and my bones, lonely, my self pity reeking with revenge for this hour to be more than it was.

Something in the night shook like a chain. I am near the end of the parking lot when I stop, glance into the dark beyond the light poles where a man is weaving toward me, walking from the fence near the old building not far away. I wonder why he hadn't simply walked through the main gate since no one was there, and why, as I hesitated, he continues to move my direction. "Heya," he said. "You!"

The muffled sound of breaking glass shattered the calm, followed by a short cry. "No!"

The man dropped to his knees, called to me, arms wild. "Over here, God! Help me!"

I move closer a few steps, see the small paper sack leaking near his knees. "I'm not God," I say. "I can't help you."

His eyes are pitiful, pleading, confused, filled with tears, and he is drooling.

"You are God. God damn you!"

"I'm not God."

"If you're not God then why can you just leave? Who gave you permission? Why do I have to come back? You must be God. Please, please, please help me, God, God Damn you."

"I can't help you." I turn my back, continue toward the main gate, look over my shoulder to make sure he isn't staggering after me with more of his drunken gibberish bullshit.

He is gone. I will never become like him.

I walked down the hill toward the train shacks, spotted a liquor store not far away, went inside, dared the clerk in my mind, and with my eyes cold and superior, not to refuse my request for a pint of booze, paid for it and left.

I slugged down a long drink, then a second and the third.

REGINA'S RECORD

Sailor hats were bouncing in the night, and a group of men and women were laughing. Two Waves asked if I would like to party with them in Milwaukee. I told them I had to get back to Minneapolis. It seemed absurd to say that to them, then I remember getting on the electric train, taking another drink when no one was looking. Someone had a transistor. Peter and Gordon were singing: *"Leaves swaying in the summer breeze, showing off their silver leaves as we walk by–"*.

And the next scene shook me with perfect clarity.

I am on my knees behind thick velvet curtains inside a confessional. I must have stopped off in Milwaukee, I'm thinking, found a church, came inside for comfort and contemplation. The priest's voice is stern, and he seems steamed about something, mentions Halloween of all things, and he says there is nothing funny about not knowing and adds that he has repeated himself to me several times, and he will say this one more time for my benefit. "The thing you *must* do, young man, is tell your grandmother where you are, that you're okay, and then you need to get the hell out of Miami as quickly as you can and go home."

Walter Reed Army Hospital

"Is there a history of mental illness in your family?"
"No."
"Do you think you need psychiatric counseling at this time?"
"No."

Walter Reed Army Hospital's psychiatric unit for enlisted men stands half a block behind the mass of old and newer buildings clustered together like a tiny city without space to grow. On the south side of the two story, vanilla brick building that houses the patients a large tree shadows the narrow strip of lawn that slopes to the sidewalk.

It is late August, ten months since I'd visited Regina in North Chicago. I had no idea that I was following in her footsteps on a timeline similar to her final days in the military.

Carl Arsalanian, a thirty-five year old Spec 5 lifer, was driving a two-star General through the Lincoln tunnel in New York City when the car stalled. Arsalanian felt panic, paralyzed with a nameless fear, he said. He couldn't move his eyelids. His hands were locked to the steering wheel. He heard everything, felt everything, but could not move.

One week after I'd been released from the closed ward on second floor, I met Arsalanian in the open ward Day Room. When it wasn't raining or we weren't scheduled for some activity, we took up chairs on the side lawn during lazy afternoons. We spoke of our lives and our troubles.

Arsalanian, a short, dark haired man with dark brown laughing eyes and a good sense of humor, called me "Yimmy" – the same way Ted had back at the old creamery house. Arsalanian was a good listener and I found his kindness and patience attractive and comforting.

I had told him about visiting my mother in North Chicago, getting drunk, ending up in Miami not sure how I got there only to find a one-way bus ticket in my jacket pocket, and nothing in my wallet. I didn't return to the University or the fraternity house where I'd been living as an eighteen-year-old freshman. Instead I hitched a ride north to Columbia, South Carolina, walked the lonely streets for a day, and slept exhausted under a tree by the State capitol that night. In the morning, with no more than five minutes of thought based on what had been dictated by my stomach, I went into a recruiting station on main street, joined the Army. After the reality of the Reception Station in nearby Ft. Jackson – followed by eight weeks in tent city during Basic Training, two weeks Leadership School, and eight weeks Advanced Infantry Training, my orders came through for the "Old Guard" in historic Ft. Myer, Virginia, behind Arlington National Cemetery. Most of the others who were regular Army in my company went to Vietnam, but because I happened to meet the six-foot minimum height requirement for ceremonial duty the DC orders took priority. Within a month, I was strutting with the others in my company, gliding in rigid perfection through various details at important places, struck by the magnitude of each event, doing exactly and precisely what I was trained to do. Elegant patent leather flawlessness in a blue uniform, white shirt, black tie, two inch heels with side-cleats to strike in unified thunder.

What I did not, could not understand, is that five minutes of childhood trauma, whenever and wherever it happens, equals a lifetime of doubt, and the doubts and fears had become more and more frequent. Acts of kindness turned into suspicion. Common talk became boring and insignificant. Duty turned to dread. Honest compliments were received and viewed through a distortion perceived as weakness in others who obviously lacked sound judgment. Rumor became fact. "No" was a challenge. "Yes" was the inner disappointment that success could be so easy. Guilt loomed everywhere. The insignificant was magnified. What was important was feared and reduced to the unimportant. Excuses became reasons. Misery was everywhere. No one cared.

I believed and had no other choice to believe that my own feelings of worthlessness had a connection with seeing Regina in Downey. Her words had locked in my head like echoes that found endless chambers. "I don't have a son. Who are you?" I couldn't connect the recent past with the distant past, didn't even think about it. The link wasn't made that the violence at the old creamery house some thirteen years earlier was the root cause of my fear of failure and until it was, I was doomed to feel sorry for myself. The more I felt sorry for myself the more I felt different, and the more I felt different the more I hoped to conform to the spirit of my fellows. Since I believed no one had suffered the way I had suffered, the worse I felt and the more I compared myself to others. And the more that happened, the more I found the need to secretly stand apart, reinvent my insides as unique and deserving without any revealing change on the outside that would make me stand out.

I wanted to show others that I was worthy as a human being, a man, and a soldier, and when those brief moments came to pass, when someone said I had done well, I didn't believe it for ten seconds. I pretended indifference when I was outraged. I lacked the ability to say no and mean no, stand up for myself, accept my own skin and who was in it –

defects and all. At the same time I wanted to apologize for something and I wasn't sure what it was or whom I should apologize to. I wanted to explain without knowing what it was that needed explanation.

At nineteen, standing along red carpets near some of the most powerful men on earth, walking near the very monuments of history that I had studied as a child, I considered myself a complete and total failure.

Invisible wounds left untreated, at least for me, had become far more dangerous than the possibility of being stabbed in the stomach with a rusty bayonet. I wanted to – but could not – peel back the layers of my own misery, confess to someone that I belonged in a nut house like my mother, tell someone that something was wrong and I desperately needed help to find out what it was, stop my head committee of whining complaints, stop the inner ongoing chorus of I, I, I, and me, me, me cloaked in outward kindness motivated by shapeless, nameless, unquenchable, ongoing fear that wore me down day after day, every day for months. Until early one weekday morning, three officers on their way to Bible study, before their work day at the Pentagon, found me curled up on a bed of needles under a wide pine tree behind the Post Chapel. I crawled out from where I was, stood at attention, saluted, told the officers who I was, and that I wasn't sure where I'd been, how long I'd been gone, and how I got there.

"Lost track of a few days, Sir," I said.

"How many?" one officer asked.

"Don't know," I answered.

Some of it came back, and some of it didn't.

Twenty-nine days earlier I'd opened my eyes to find myself curled around a toy shovel in a tractor tire at one end of the parade field. I was horrified that someone would find out, relieved when they didn't. The next day or the next I was talking to some bow legged kid named Billy. He had yellow eyes. His clothes were filthy and he stunk. We met on a street in Baltimore. He said he was on his way to New York City. I didn't tell him where I'd been or that I had no idea where I was going. Hours earlier, almost like a sweatless zombie, I had walked out of the main gate at Ft. Myer. There was an excitement in leaving, the thrill of risk, but those emotions were soon replaced by the hum of nothingness which is exactly the drug I wanted when I walked. And so I walked and walked and walked and walked until I met Billy going the same direction. "I'm a Navy deserter," he said openly. "Two years been living from one Salvation Army to the next."

We caught a ride with someone then someone else. Billy and I parted company somewhere in New York City and I thought it was because we had stopped walking and started thinking. He was headed for the Bowery, he said, and I couldn't make up my busy mind whether or not to go along so he left and I continued walking and called it destiny that had we separated. I moved into my walking mode again, hoped for the mind-numb, the thoughtless blank where the world and its people disappear and are no longer dangerous. I believed that if I walked far enough and long enough I could finally sleep and dream of home, and when I woke up I would have money in my pocket and everything would be different and I would, by magic, become normal.

As darkness fell, I took a chance and asked a street cop for directions. "Get the fuck out of here," he shouted.

I was crushed by the experience, walked for hours, walked until I found a two ton army truck behind the National Guard Armory in Queens, curled up on the dust covered front seat, said an Act of Contrition, prayed for sleep; certain men were hunting me and when I was captured these faceless men would deny me sleep, forever. I worried all night about these men, listened for their footsteps. What would happen if they found me? What tribunal would try me for my sins? Would I have to confess? Yes, I would say, I am guilty. Yes, I don't believe in God the Father, God the Son, or God the Holy Ghost. I believe in Henry Aaron and the head of the Joint Chiefs of Staff, and my grandmother.

My friend Arsalanian seemed to understand my stories, promise he wouldn't repeat them. "Some of us have to figure out why we feel different, Yimmy," he said. "You won't be able to live good until you do."

> "This young soldier, who does not appear ill and has no complaints, apparently suffers from an emotional disorder not clearly defined but manifesting itself in a tendency to sleep for extended periods. In recent weeks, according to his intake officer, he has shown periods of emotional lability and discomfort. According to his Commanding Officer, Captain Marfield, soldier had been unacounted for by officers and staff at Headquarters. Co. Ft. Myer, VA for a period of 28 days AWOL. Soldier indicated upon admission that he left KP one afternoon, and began walking 'somewhere north'. He stated he wasn't certain what brought on this behavior but that he was 'extremely tired and had a lot of strange thoughts' and felt that walking would clear his mind. When questioned, soldier would not elaborate as to what his thinking was or what prompted his action to leave the base and not return for the 28-day period lost. According to soldier, he traveled to Queens, New York and entered the World's Fair without paying. He stated that he had seen the Pieta in the Vatican

Pavilion but had no feeling toward this event or what he had seen, and could not understand why. During interview, soldier was asked where he was during the remainder of the 28-day period in question. He did not offer any further explanation except to state that he has had some brief periods of time where he does not recall events. When asked if he had ever abused alcohol or drugs, soldier responded: 'Never had drugs. And I don't think I drink anymore than anyone else'. There are no clear previous demonstrations of any specific difficulty or tendencies toward abnormal behavior. This physician spoke with Staff Sergeant Bayle, soldier's NCO. Sergeant Bayle stated that soldier performed duties well at various ceremonial functions in the DC and Arlington, VA area and there were no signs of difficulty. The only single clear indication of distress in not accepting the reality in which he currently finds himself is that he has recently avoided his military responsibilities by leaving his regular duty station. Diagnosis at this time undetermined. General prognosis good. Observe."

Captain M. Gellan, MD
Walter Reed Psychiatric Section

Hennepin County General Hospital
Psychiatric Ward

"At around 1:30 a.m., Minneapolis police officers brought in a 21 year old white male following an emergency call to an apartment in the city. Patient's room mate reported finding him in bed *passed out and bleeding from numerous razor cuts to both wrists. Patient's room mate told officers that patient had recently been discharged from military service and had been drinking. Patient appears in good physical health and his vital signs are good. He is intoxicated at this hour but remains cooperative. The cuts have been sutured. When asked the reasons for his actions, patient said he'd made a mistake and it wouldn't happen again and that he 'was sorry for causing any trouble'. When it was suggested he seek further evaluation in a Veterans' hospital patient said: 'Not a chance'. When asked if he would care to remain in this hospital for a short period to undergo an evaluation he refused and signed himself out AMA."*

Charles O'Brian, RN

Like Mother, Like Son

The leaves had just started to turn when I went out pretending to kill myself for the second time, to bring attention again to my arms where I hoped self pity would bleed itself out and leave me alone. I was working the night shift in a car coat factory, quit for another job then another job and one more the next week. I had a girlfriend. She was in college. I told her about my mother. She listened and seemed to understand. There was music. Ed Ames and his cup runneth over with love.

I got a construction job. I traveled with a crew of hard ass fanatics to South Dakota. I was tar man on a dorm roof. I had a drink of cheap beer one night and then another and who counts anyway because I was spinning into something dark and foreboding. When I opened my eyes into an impossible light, three men and a woman were standing over me.

"Why did you do this, son?" someone asked.

Thirty-six stitches on my left arm and twenty-two on my right.

"We're taking him to jail for safekeeping," someone said.

My three cellmates have two final requests before my transfer to the St. Cloud VA this morning. Hold the *Life Magazine* cover (which had been fashioned into a funnel) very still while the guy in the cell block upstairs pours fermented pear juice down through a floor crack into our cups.

Nothing about this is easy. I climb half way up the bars, my bandaged left arm outstretched, with my hand around the tapered end of the paper cone while one of the other prisoners stands directly below the cone's spout, waiting for the stream. We fill four cups that way, then toast the genius of our anonymous benefactor. The second request is easy. Stand at the far end of the walkway with a mop handle offered as a makeshift rifle, and go through the exact ceremony of a guard walking the Tomb of the Unknown Soldier in Arlington.

My motion is fluid and perfect, ten steps short of the twenty-one needed over the flat black mat, but I make the adjustment. My mop handle rests at right shoulder arms, away from the inner cell bars at all times. I stop sharp with my left heel moving outward to close with my right, at the same time moving right shoulder arms to port arms, waiting twenty-one seconds, turning sharp, heel to toe turn, twenty-one seconds again, left shoulder arms, smart, stiff, twenty-one seconds again and I'm into my strut, my puppet walk, my gliding elegance only to stop again, snap my electric heels together, make the metal heel shanks rivet the crowd in a stunning display of perfected patriotism. The Tomb is a place of importance, I tell my cellmates. Even hippies who wander there stand quiet. West Pointers drool. No jokes. There is something about the place. People don't even cough loud.

My cellmates applaud. "You ain't a fuckin' queer or nothin' are you?" one of them asks.

Ten minutes later I am led out of the cellblock, cuffed, escorted from the building to the back seat of an unmarked squad car. The two deputies chat with one another, smoke, complain about having to make a long drive on such a nice day. Around noon we stop at a fast food place to use the rest room and order burgers to go. They bring me inside to a line of frightened people who quickly allow us to the counter, avoid me as if I were a dead cat. I am embarrassed. I feel sorry for the frightened children, their parents bending, whispering in their little ears that I'm someone who has been bad.

I am wearing my Milwaukee Braves baseball cap, a warm-up shirt with red sleeves, my army fatigue jacket, jeans, brown boots, handcuffs. I don't think it is proper to smile in handcuffs, and I don't.

Two and half hours later we make the turn onto a long dark road lined with large trees blocking all but a few rays of afternoon sunlight. A couple of old men are walking on the shoulder with hands behind their backs, hunched like umpires, staring at some distant point beyond nothingness.

The tennis court has no net. There is a water tower and what looks like a power plant and a green house with missing panes replaced here and there with plywood. The three story buildings seem endless, each connected to the other and each exactly the same, fronted by white rock around bushes trimmed neat by some fanatic. Each section of buildings has a wide courtyard and a set of steps. There are bars on all of the third floor windows. I wonder about those bars. I wonder what will happen next, happen inside the buildings. Those thoughts overwhelm all other thoughts.

We park in the back of one of the buildings. The deputies walk along side of me as we take the steps up to Admissions where a man behind a desk puts down his newspaper and stands. One of the deputies hands the man a file folder while the other brings out a key and unlocks the cuffs. The man unlocking the cuffs is as close to me as he has ever been, the top of his head near my chest. He says something as he releases my hands. I didn't hear what he said. He asks me if I heard him. "No," I say. "I didn't hear." He says, "Then you better listen next time. I said that you're going to be here a long time, boy."

"Fuck you," I say.

"What did you say to me?"

"I said, fuck you."

He drove his left shoulder into mine, but not hard. More like a childish act of provocation as he passed. Without thinking I jabbed my left elbow in his lower back, hard. He groaned and straightened, held his side, turned, his eyes filled with rage, his face pale with anger as his leather pistol belt squeaked from his effort to move toward me. He took one or two steps then stopped when his partner called his name, coaxed him away. He retreated, shook his head, too proud it seemed to rub the sore in his back, mumbling something about retards as the two went out the door, replaced at almost the same moment by two fat aides, both with black belts jangling keys announcing their arrival.

"You aren't going to give us trouble are you?" one of them asked, smiling.

"No trouble," I replied.

We move out into a long hallway tunnel where a man on a golf cart hums past with Bozo hair pushed back wild from the speed. We walk past a large chow hall. The hallway slopes there, past a canteen, past a chapel, around a corner past another chow hall, past a small library, through a dark door, up a flight of stairs, then another, the keys rattle and the door opens. We're in a hallway, men are standing, smoking, and one says, "Are you the new rutabaga king? Are you the slave kid, shit bird with interstate slick?"

A nurse steps out of a small office and looks at me. Another nurse accidentally bumps her from behind trying to catch a look. "He's so young," the first nurse says.

The aides motion me to the Day Room. A tall man in the latrine is combing his hair, his penis limp in the sink. There is a hairless recess on his skull.

In the Day Room, near the nurses' station, someone has turned up the volume on a radio. Patsy Cline is singing. I've heard Patsy Cline before.

A patient in pajamas and a blue robe passes me, close, and our eyes meet.

"You better find another better way to get yourself home, boy," he says. "This is a hospital for crazy people."

St. Cloud Veterans Administration Hospital

> "This twenty-one year old, six foot tall, 165-lb. veteran was admitted this hour with no complaints. He is a transfer from the county jail in Brookings, South Dakota. He appears in good physical condition. He is aware of date and year. He was court ordered here for further evaluation after an apparent suicide attempt. According to court documents he was working for a construction company and walked away from his job after a disagreement with his foreman. Brookings authorities were later notified by a local hospital that he had slashed his arms and was admitted to their emergency room for sutures. Gauze on both arms was removed by this physician and further examination revealed numerous sutures from his elbows to his wrists. When asked what prompted his actions, veteran stated that he wasn't certain, but that he'd had thoughts about his mother. He admitted alcohol consumption. Telephone contact was made with his grandmother. Mrs. Van Amber stated that her youngest daughter (veteran's mother) is a long term VA patient at Downey VA. She went on to say that before her grandson dropped out of the University and joined the Service he had gone to visit his mother and the visit had affected him in an adverse way, but she could not elaborate. His grandmother also stated

> *that she had some few typical problems with him growing up, but none were severe and that he is a good boy. Diagnosis at this time is offered: Schizophrenic reaction, moderate. Suicide risk. Closed ward supervision. No privileges. Observe."*
>
> W Nelson, MD

Most violence, I've come to know from talking with others who have worked in psychiatric hospitals, does not often come under outside scrutiny, and the VA system, once the largest psychiatric system on earth, is no different. And while some incidents were, I suppose, officially documented when there were obvious injuries, the first assault I witnessed could not have been reported because no aides were present to write anything down, and who is going to believe someone who is crazy anyway?

What erupted those first days after I was on the wards was not on C floor where I'd been assigned, but in the post chapel where a group of men – most around twenty-five years older than myself – had gathered for Sunday services, led there by two chubby aides through the labyrinth of dull stairways and long tunnels. The aides escaped the boredom of church by stationing themselves outside the chapel while the rest of us, several from other parts of the hospital, were waiting for Mass to begin. I am speaking now of men broken by the shock of war, serious accidents, genetic fate, some unspeakable calamity – patients who saw fit to join the celebration of prayer, a few who had that same whitish, six inch sunken area on the upper side of their skulls, humans that, it seemed to me, didn't know the difference between a song book and a salt shaker. But we were there, and I was there, convicting myself again for the stupidity of getting into something I sensed was not going to be easy to get out of.

The priest had come out, a stocky man with a stern face that appeared in need of a blood transfusion. He made his important genuflect in front of the altar, moved behind it and glanced to the morning gathering. As soon as he spoke, a man, two rows deep in the middle section of pews, responded loudly in some indecipherable way, rambling on about Jesus and Mary and Joseph, and I forget what else.

The priest paid no attention at first, and went on with his ritual. Within a few seconds, he was interrupted again by another outburst this time from someone else in the gathering. Near the back, a man had raised his voice, spoke about "wages and sin and not getting paid" and at almost the same time, behind me and off to my left, came an odd but distinct sound I had heard everywhere except inside a church. The click-chink of a cigarette lighter being flicked open. I turned to the sound, distracted for a moment by the first man who was uttering something else and the second who was going on and on, still with his strange topic. In that pew behind me, a tall, dark haired man in street clothes held the lighter. He had a cigarette firm between his lips – and was about to strike the flint, then did. By this time the priest was running from the altar in the aisle along the middle pews, his eyes murderously explosive, glaring at the first man who had interrupted him, pushing aside three or four who stood in his way until he reached the poor patient, grabbed him by his pyjama shirt, and slapped him across his face. "I've told you and told you and told you. No interruptions!"

This poor patient cowered, covering his face from further attack while the others, including myself, stood shocked by what the priest had just done.

"I want my wages!" the man near the back called out. "Pay me!"

The priest couldn't get to the back of the pews fast enough.

When he did there was a second struggle to get past the line of men blocking his movement through the pew and the priest, apparently not overly concerned which patient should suffer from his wrath, struck the wrong man, slapping him on top of his head three or four times, shouting, "I won't have this. I won't have this. This is God's house! I won't have it!"

As he was retreating up the aisle toward the altar, his eyes burning with heated disgust, he suddenly spotted the man behind me who by now was smoking freely, in a deliberately exaggerated manner, drawing rapid puffs of smoke from his cigarette, blowing little smoke rings that rose up one after another toward the high ceiling, and each time extending his hand out about two feet before he drew in another rapid set of puffs, blew more rings, all seemingly with the idea of drawing attention to his own irreverence, undaunted by the priest's furious approach.

By the look of utter disbelief on the priest's face, I honestly thought he was going to explode a third time, throw himself over the pews at the man, and beat him senseless. I think he might have done if the man hadn't stopped him, and I mean right now, with the loudest, deepest, most chilling voice I have ever heard. "If–you–come–any–closer, Father, I–will–kill–you."

The priest drew back like a frightened child, completely and suddenly powerless as if he'd seen the face of Christ in this man or was staring into the very eyes of Satan and wasn't sure whether to kneel or run. Without saying more, the priest moved back up to the altar, made his genuflect, and walked out of the rear of the chapel without saying another word.

For a minute or two, standing in that chapel among these men – some sad and confused, some gravely ill and shaking out of control, a few looking to others for a sign of what to do next – I felt a brotherhood of the spirit, a kind of pleasant oneness that swept away all other thoughts and feelings.

The man who was smoking moved from his pew, went to a nearby exit, shoved open the door like he meant business, and, as if he were in some pool hall and couldn't find an ashtray, flicked his cigarette outside, spat in the same direction, came back inside, and left the same way we had all entered.

As we filed out of the chapel not far behind the man, I overheard one of the aides say that services were getting shorter and shorter these days.

I looked for the man, thought about what he did, privately chuckled over it, wanted to learn more about him and where he got the power to do such a thing, why he was here and where he came from, and how long he'd been here.

I didn't see him again.

I spent five months on the closed ward. Bing Crosby's *White Christmas* played on the Day Room radio on Christmas Eve. I missed my grandmother, tried to sleep through it, to dream.

A week later, soon after the New Year, several college women from a nearby University came on the ward for a dance in the Day Room. One patient, a short little man named Wayne (who slept in the bunk next to mine) reminded me of pictures I'd seen of General Douglas MacArthur except Wayne had no teeth. He was someone I had liked, not in a perverse way because he was ill, but in the way that he didn't make any sense, seemed completely harmless, laughed a lot at nothing, told me that he had founded the Interstate Highway system and made the government "use old postage stamps and spider shit for a roadbed". He always managed to seek me out in the chow hall, gorge his mouth with frozen butter and ooze it between his lips, licking on his morning toast. "Want some?" he asked.

During a slow dance with one young woman, Wayne reached down his pajama pants and began masturbating. The aides weren't watching and the girl pretended not to notice, but before Wayne ejaculated, he ran full speed toward the latrine, slid past it in his cloth slippers, and retreated with his legs running almost in place, shouting "Wheeeeeeee!"

At the time, I thought his actions were hilarious and certainly harmless, not fully understanding that psychiatry seems to frown upon acting out such fantasies, or lack of control, on the ward. Early the next day Wayne was not in his bunk when I awoke, and didn't take his place in the morning chow line. Aides told me he was transferred to another ward.

During those first weeks there were tests and more tests. EEG, MMPI, Mr. Rorschach and his bug-doodles, subtracting from a hundred by sevens, and others. Once Dr. Nelson, the ward psychiatrist, learned about Regina, I suddenly had the attention of two psychologists and two psychiatrists – all wanting to play chess and chat, apparently interested in what I had to say about things, how I said them and why. "What do you mean by that? What makes you say that? What do you think about that? Where do you expect to be in five years? Why this and why that, and why not this or that or that?

These were kind inquiries, but not very helpful since it was obvious they were veiled with an agenda.

After three months of boring visits to Occupational Therapy and Physical Therapy and a small swimming pool someone usually defecated in, I wanted out, didn't wait until someone gave me permission, and on my way up the stairs from the chow hall one night in mid-winter, found an outside door slightly ajar. With the aides momentarily out of sight below and behind me, I slipped outside into the shocking night. Twenty below zero, but the wind behind me. I had on blue jeans, an undershirt, long sleeved shirt, socks, tennis shoes, and a thin blue nylon baseball warm-up jacket that means nothing in winter. I ran around half the length of the hospital to get to the front, ran through snow banks and across the icy roads and finally down the long main road the deputies had brought me in on three months earlier, ran five miles without stopping until I got downtown where I carded in one liquor store, refused service. I stopped this college student on the frozen sidewalk, gave him what money I had in my pocket (four dollars I think it was), pleaded with him to buy me a pint of anything labeled Southern Comfort and he did and I drank it, and the night warmed and the wind was nothing.

I like the Righteous Brothers. Words rising above the wind. *"Soul and Inspiration. All I've got...."* something and something about being brave in love. I don't want to be a coward. I'm a rebel and I'll never be understood. I want to stay downtown, listen to the *"music of the traffic in the city, linger on the sidewalks were the neon lights are pretty"*, be the leader of the pack, walk the talk like the guy in the chapel who blew smoke rings in church, didn't take shit from anyone. I want someone to save the last dance for me, become Mister Tambourine Man – play a song for you, pick up the pieces when somebody steals your heart, play solitaire until dawn, become the lawn mower, the steam roller, the loco-motion, the Man Who Shot Liberty Valance. Somebody, anybody. Not me.

In my head swim I thought about hitchhiking home, then decided against it because my grandmother would wonder about my late arrival, worry about making sense of the story I'd tell her. And I was certain the police were looking for me, Dr. Richard Kimble, the fugitive wrongly accused, on the road, cold and lonely in a dark strange place belting out

Righteous Brothers songs, loud and louder.

A frosty squad car passed, and I felt panic.

I wasn't sure what to do next so I walked the five miles back to the hospital, a place where I believed I would never get free from again, listened as my shoes crackled on the crisp snow, faced the biting wind on my face, stinging as the booze wore off, then running, stopping, gagging, running again down the long tree lined driveway until I moved inside to the warmth of the main lobby, turning myself into the night clerk who looked at me with both eyes, shook her head, and said: "You wait over there and don't go anywhere."

The two aides who came to take me back to the ward laughed as they approached, told me they had no idea I was gone.

The next morning Dr. Nelson met me in the nurses' station, told me that whatever I thought I suffered from was not the same as what my mother suffered, and it was immature to pull a stunt like I had pulled, and went on to say that should I try something again he would consider medications to settle me down.

Two months passed – months of OT and PT and group therapy and visits from my girlfriend and my grandmother, their eyes filled with concern. I apologized for bringing heartache, promised to do better.

Stand up and be a man, I told myself. Will power. Hitch my wagon to a star.

Finally, in mid-March, after meeting with staff, trying to convince them I would behave myself, wasn't insane, would get a job, reform, shape up my life, I was given a discharge with a strong suggestion to find work.

❖

Two days before I was released a nurse approached me in the Day Room asked me to follow her, took me into a room off the ward where she handed me a blanket, told me to lay on the bunk and cover myself because she was going to give me a shot that would make me very cold, and then, a short time later, very hot. I asked her why she was giving me this shot. She said the doctor had ordered it, wanted to "find out something". I asked her what it was she was giving me. "It won't hurt," she said.

I was a fool for allowing her to administer that hypo without more information, but I wanted out and was willing to do almost anything for that to happen.

My body was ravaged by cold chills shortly followed by heat enough to make me sweat and that was it – nothing more.

After Regina's records came, I requested my own files from three separate institutions. Two dozen pages from the VA and no mention about the hypo. It didn't much matter. I had done far worse outside the VA. And, anyway, they could always say I was crazy.

At noon, with March snow still banked high in the courtyard, my girlfriend picked me up in her Galaxy 500, told me in soft words that she didn't want to upset me on the ward, but now that I was out, she needed to tell me that she was pregnant, beginning to show a lot, and what did I want to do?

"Get married," I said, "I suppose."

"Okay," she said.

It is March 15, 1971, night. I am standing inside the main gate at Downey VA in North Chicago within sight of Building 131. My wife doesn't know where I am. My grandmother doesn't know where I am. And for three or four days I wasn't always sure exactly where I was and didn't care, and then I was sure where I was and wanted to care but couldn't care much without twenty drinks.

Inside the small security and information building I deliberately avoided stepping too close to the counter, stood back a little to avoid the stoic woman with puffy hair who might get a whiff of alcohol and sweat on my pores, in my clothes, on my breath.

I had been riding the trains back and forth between Milwaukee and Chicago all day and into the evening, stopping at Great Lakes for the walk up the big hill, but not getting off, riding for two or three or four days trying to get my mind clear – make things strong in order to see Regina, powerful enough to take anything she said or didn't say and laugh about it later or smile at her or nod without consequences – take it with a grain of salt, drinking in my strength to prepare, guzzling and gulping to bring about and capture and sustain my love for her, my deepest pure emotions.

When the trains stopped running for the night, I found a cheap hotel in Waukeegan not sure whether I should kill myself or go bowling. I paced the floor unable to leave, unable to sleep safe in good dreams, fearful of fear, uncertain about what to do next but hoping the committee in my head would stop reminding me that my stomach was turning to cardboard and cardboard doesn't do well in the rain, or in dank basements where it rots, or in the damp night chilled by unstoppable stale air.

Drinking toward oblivion without moving beyond courage is a trick not easy to master, but when it works it makes earth people tolerable and the others right. The swelling rise of rum in my brain sets me on the high road, allows an evenness between elation and depression, brings back the lost magic of wonder and awe, that certain specific place where all that dwells bad becomes good, tolerable, decent, laughable, stupid.

❖

The clerk tells me that Regina has been moved to a VA hospital in Tomah, Wisconsin and I missed her by only days. I said, "Oh, that's all right," and, I added, "Weather is chilly for this time of year. It goes right through a person doesn't it?"

The parking lot between Buildings 131 and 100 is darkened, and I'm standing smoking, gazing to the lighted windows above. I'm not sure what came over me, self-pity again maybe, but I fell to my knees in the darkness there, said, "Oh God. Oh God Oh God."

I'll need to figure out a way to explain again. Come up with a story. Mend fences. Make it right back home. I'll tell my wife that it's time we all start going to Mass again. I'll tell her that the reason I didn't take my shaving kit or suitcase is that I thought I'd only be gone for the day and I couldn't call because something came up, an emergency – the death of a friend's baby. "It was tragic," I'll say. "And during the funeral someone else became deathly ill and I was at their bedside."

I'll go on and on until she his convinced that I am not crazy. I have been explaining all of my life.

After I left Downey that night and took the train again to Chicago, I bought a bus ticket for Sioux Falls, South Dakota, sucked down a few more drinks in the rest room, boarded the bus, sat next to a young woman who slipped me a handful of green pills, showed me her lower tummy tattoo, said this trip would be all right. I fell asleep or passed out, and woke up in the train station in Fargo, North Dakota. We live in Omaha. I had told my wife that things would be better in Omaha. The beer is stronger in Nebraska.

REGINA'S RECORD

Regina is Crying.

Elavil, Proketazine, Cascara, Thorazine,
    Trihexyphenidyl,
Sparine, hallucinations, shakiness, Fluphenazine,
    Reserpine, Compazine, Stelazine, dizziness,
Stelazine in coffee,
    Phenelzine, fainting, talking to no one in
    particular, Vioform
Tripelennamine, Melleril, Prolixin, drooling,
    Artane, Calamine Lotion, Emesis and loose
stools, more vomiting.
Nafcillin, Cortiforte, Carphenazine Maleate, fainted.
    Demazin, hot soaks, Synalar Cream, Permitil,
Haldol, nightmares,
Bromphemiramine and phenylephrine and
    phenylpropanolamine.

    *"Crying all through this a.m.. Possible Med.
reaction."*

Hydrocortisone, Thiamine, Niacinamide, Tofranil,
    rash, insomnia,
Tetracycline, Coal Tar, shuffling, Frisofulvin,
    Pecatal, Temaril, Triancinone, confusion,
Ivory soap, Emesis and loose stools. Mood changes,
    inflammation on buttocks the size of a
    fifty-cent piece.

Neomycin and Dexamethasone, Nystatin Ointment,
    band aid, headache, chest hurts, heartache,
Zincon shampoo, Desenex
    Sodium Amytal, trembling, shaking,
    walks funny.

    "Walked into door and bumped her head.
    Check meds."

Serpasil, Valium, Librium, Dalmane, Navane,
Sinequan, Docusate Sodium, Halotex, Metronidazole,
Orenzyme, Acetaminophen, Vitamin C,
    Emesis and loose stools, vomiting.

    "Fell in Day Room. Possible Med. reaction.
    Check charts."

Ace bandage, Penicillin, Heating Pad, Maalox,
    Phisohex, itch, Erythromycin,
Light Kling dressing, Dermatitis, Mineral oil,
    lanolin acid glycerin, Gantrisin, Carisoprodol,
Psoriasis, scratching,
Micatin, Propylene Glycol, Maalox, stomach ache,
    vomit, Vitamins A, D, B1, B2,
B3, C,

    "While in full bed restraints this p.m., her
body turned a light blue in color, and she has an
extremely foul odor. Nurses and aides are
gagging. OD called. Taken to isolation. OD is
checking meds."

REGINA'S RECORD

    Cogentin, Folic Acid daily, confusion,
        drowsiness, jerkiness,
        Emesis and loose stools, vomiting.
        Cold Compress, Lindane, Septra,
Ampicillin, Lotrimin, Mycelex,
Mercurochrome, warm water, Parkinsonian walk,
        Emesis and loose stools, vomiting.

    "Regina is crying. Check meds."

Tylenol, Emesis and loose stools. Light sensitive,
        blurred vision, tunnel vision,
Bactrim, chest pain, dry mouth, sore throat,
Flagyl, Emesis and loose stools, vomiting.
        Feosal, Hyoscine, Warm Compresses,
        Orange Juice, a beer, Pall Mall straights,
        ceiling smoke,
Doxidan, Colace, Emesis and loose stools, vomiting.
Aspirin, salt and pepper in coffee,
        Emesis and loose stools, asbestos
        vomiting, constipation, diarrhea, nausea.

    "Walked into wall. Check meds."

    "Patient passing out on elevator on way
    to breakfast. Indigestion.
    Patient passed out on floor.
    Urinary retention.
    Patient in hallway
    passed out."

Fungus, lethargy, open sores, menstrual cramps,
        loss of appetite, jaundice,
Dark urine, Myopic, milking her breasts.

"Asked why she didn't eat her toast. She said she didn't eat anything with the letter 'T' in it."

Vaginal irritation, infection, Lordosis, lacerated cervix, muscle spasms, numbness, thready pulse, irregular heart beat, adrenaline, abortion.

"Patient Van Amber's med. chart mixed with Linda Collins' med. chart."

"This patient is badly in need of personality and social adjustment. She smokes heavily, drinks alcoholic beverages, not addicted to any habit forming drugs."
I. Corcanus, MD

Overdosed four times per day on Reserpine from July 22, 1957 to July 26.

Overdosed four times per day with Reserpine from August 26 to August 28, 1958.

Overdosed continuously on Prolixin from August 1, 1962 to September 24, 1965.

On March 11, 1971, the VA transferred Regina to Tomah VA in western Wisconsin. A ward for women had opened there, and officials stated she would be closer to relatives. Regina, of course, had no choice in the matter even though she had pleaded with the staff to let her stay. The nurses poked her into a halcyon state with Demerol, then escorted her off the ward to a car in the parking lot outside Building 131. A female aide drove her out the main gate, turned west, and began the four hour drive to the place that had rejected her nineteen years earlier.

> "Admission from Downey VAH [at] 2:30 p.m. Seems to be sociable. Stated she and the aide stopped for a few beers, and said: 'There is nothing you can do about it.' Says she has never been married. Very cooperative. Cheerful disposition. Placed on closed ward."
>
> Patricia Gertasen, RN

> "This new admission would only answer questions with yes or no this evening. No cheerful disposition displayed."
>
> Julie Thorseth, SN

> "Miss Van Amber, 48 years of age, one-hundred percent service connected for a psychiatric disorder was transferred here from Downey on March 11 of this year. This patient was described in childhood as a nail-biting, temper prone person. She was also bashful and said to have been tolerated by her classmates. She was also described as an introvert. She did not finish high school in the 4 years but had to repeat and did finish after 5 years as 108 in a class of 146. She

was described as never having been a leader i n any respect. The writer feels that this patient could improve gradually in the hospital setting here. The diagnosis of schizophrenic reaction, severe, paranoid type is offered. Although this diagnosis does not conform with that most recently given, namely chronic undifferentiated type, I feel that since the patient is hallucinating periodically and does manifest delusional ideation in various forms, that the paranoiac elements should be identified."

Arthur M. Deal, MD

"Patient was very friendly this morning. After dinner was allowed to nap for 1 hour. Was given a smoke."

Julie Thorseth, SN

"Received by mail package from Downey containing 1 dress."

Karen Torberg, SN

"Patient escorted to Central Linen this a.m. by another woman patient. Seemed quite willing to be able to work. Stacked towels in a fast way. Not bad for an old lady."

Jeannette Paskell, LPN

"Central Linen refuses to take her back because of her past work record which was poor. Seems

content to sit by herself curled in chair."
                              Jeannette Paskell, LPN

"Patient Van Amber fell by her bunk this a.m. There didn't appear to be any reason for this fall. No injuries noted."
                              Karen Torberg, SN

Overdosed continuously in Tomah on Thorazine from June 5, 1973 to November 5, 1974.

Overdosed four times per day on Mellaril from February 7, 1972 to March 3, 1972, and again from November 20, 1973 to November 27, 1974, and again on April 10, 1980.

Overdosed four times per day on Stelazine from September 1, 1974 to November 21, 1974, and again from the end of August, 1979 to October 6, 1980.

> *"Numerous studies, including some by the VA, have concluded that little evidence exists to support simultaneous use of more than one psycho-therapeutic drug on the same patient – a practice commonly referred to as polypharmacy. These studies have shown that polypharmacy increases the possibility of adverse reactions and have suggested that it be avoided if possible. The more medications a patient is given, the greater risks of adverse side effects. No tests on animals have shown polypharmacy to be a safe means of treating psychosis."*
>   Comptroller General to Congress, 1975

"Regina fell over the ottoman in Tomah, fell and vomited getting up from a chair, tripped over her own feet and fell, tripped over a paper plate in the chow hall doorway. . . fell and sustained a laceration above her right eye with a contusion on the bridge of her nose. Her nose has a transverse fracture of distal 3rd nasal bone with displacement of fragment."

"Regina fell and cut her lips. Slight abrasion on her chin. Fell outside on the driveway. Received an abrasion on her left knee. She fell striking her face on pavement. Sustained a scraped nose and discolored left eye. Her left leg appears to be turned in."

Regina fell near her bunk and vomited the effects of two psychotropic medications, then three, then four, the highest dosage levels of psychotropic drugs in VA history. The experimental mixes of Stelazine, Thorazine, Mellaril, Haldol, Prolixin, Elavil, and other "anti-psychotics", made her drool, forced her onto the Day Room floor after she became too dizzy to stand, forced her to stay in a chair, forced her head one way then another, forced her tongue to stab the mean air.

She fell and vomited bile colored mucus. She fell while getting out of the van returning from the VA's main medical facility in Madison, where she had been for an examination of a tumor on her buttocks, and a previous fall. She had an injury to her right thigh on the last fall. She fell from Haldol, fell from the mix of dosages like someone drunk from a gallon of gin, Southern Comfort, rum, wine, beer – four times a day,

REGINA'S RECORD

mixed into a pail, gulped. *"She fell to the sidewalk as she took one step. Eyes very puffy."*

"She caught her foot on the leg of a chair and tripped and sprawled to floor. Swollen left wrist". She fell backwards by the nurses' station and *"had a swelling of the 1st thoracic vertebra"*. She slipped in the shower and fell, bruised her little toe. She bumped into the wall and fell. *"She fell on the stairwell going to Music Therapy"* and a couple days later the OD in Tomah decided to X-ray the swollen ankle and it revealed a fracture.

"She fell in the parking lot behind Building 400, struck her head on the curb — sustained lacerations and contusions above her left eye." "She slipped on a wet area in the Day Room as she was going to the chapel." "Fell on the way to laboratory and sustained a laceration to the lateral left eyebrow and left forehead. T h r e e sutures."

"Regina fell in the bunk area, couldn't get up right away, and her pulse was thready." She fell when a nurse was trying to help her get out of bed. *"She fell and rolled over and over on the lawn outside the building."* Then she began limping and the falling got worse. *"She fell for no apparent reason"*, tripped over her own feet for the fifth time, *"fell in front of Building 404 on her way to the Madison VA to have an eye check-up, and fractured her other ankle. She slipped on*

some spilt food in the dining hall and fell." "She fell in OT and stood with blood dripping from her gums. The left side of her face was bleeding, her eye and nose was pink colored." "She fell from a chair in PT." "She slipped on water near the stairs and fell."

She fell and knocked out a tooth, stuck her tongue out through swollen lips and showed the nurse. "My tooth," she said.

"This patient has trouble walking. Couldn't hardly walk at all. Her eye sight is possibly poor."

She fell while going out a door. Her left ankle was swollen, X-rayed, another fracture noted. *"Regina was walking back from the dining room this morning and she ran into a brick wall corner. She walks very fast. Told her not to walk so fast."*
 "She is unable to walk alone."

In the Day Room Regina slipped on urine that another patient had done, and there was "a lump on the back of her head." Two hours later, sitting in the Day Room, she suddenly clasped her chest with both hands and said, "Oh my God, pain." Patricia Gertasen, the RN, asked her where she hurt. "In my chest," she said. "My chest hurts."
 Gertasen said that Regina was "someone not good at reporting her own history".

In the chow hall, she grabbed her chest with both hands. The aide, Marie Little Wolf, asked if she'd had a chest pain. Regina said, "Yes."

"I told patient not to swallow food so fast," Little Wolf had said.

The following day she had another chest pain, and the day after she bent over in her chair clutching her chest in pain. "Probably over-medicated," wrote Little Wolf.

> "The patient's file was mixed in with Geneva Brown's file. Have meds been changed?"

> "This woman does not look where she is going because she bumped into wall. For no apparent reason this woman frequently falls or runs into things while ambulating."

> "Regina has difficulty walking. There is a lump on her outer aspect. She also has a swollen face, especially on the right side. The swelling is possibly due to sunburn or a fall."

> "She fell while walking in front of building 400 on the road. May have tripped on her pant leg as it was long and dragging on the ground."

Regina almost fell walking to the dining room again. Her face was ashen, saliva running out of her mouth. "She fell and bruised her toe" and once again when X-rays were taken the OD found a fracture. She fell backward from a rocking chair, fell in the bathroom, and fell on the floor again.

She fell by her bed attempting to sit in a chair, and the nurse noted that the fall was due to "possible med. side effects". Her right lower rib area on her back was scratched with that fall. On the next fall she struck her forehead again when she ran into a doorframe. She fell, hard. Fell on floors never meant for bones to fall on, ran into hard things that didn't move.

> "Regina Van Amber fell walking from the porch to the Day Room. She tripped on a footstool and fell face first onto the floor. Patient did not see the foot stool." She fell on the way back from bingo, hurt her face again – *"bruises over left eye and forehead".*
>
> "Wheelchair requested."

> "Fell down from wheelchair, back parking lot of Building 400. Sustained abrasions on left side of face and superficial laceration on upper lip."

> "Going to elevator Regina Van Amber tripped over dirty wash bag landing on left side hitting mouth on floor, biting tongue and upper lip. Bleeding spontaneously."

> "This patient's eyesight is poor. Request eye examination." "This patient does not want to

change beds for new arrivals." "Patient was attacked by Francis Wells this a.m.. Struck on back of neck with chair."

"Medication adjustment made by Dr. Kellen. Prolixin IM, 400 milligrams Q.I.D. [four times per day], Amytal, Haldol regular dose."

"Patient went to K-Mart with group. Behaved like a lady should!"

"Today, cholesterol was ordered on the patient because she had severe cholesterol accumulation on the Lasix. She smiled this morning for the first time in long time."

"She is quiet, withdrawn, shy, does not associate with anybody, doesn't talk. For the last two weeks she says hello from time to time, but is otherwise very shy and frightful. She has periods where she gets very mad and doesn't socialize with anybody for several days. Otherwise, her condition seems to be improving."

"Patient doesn't look you straight in the eyes most of the time. She answers questions by bending her head that she is doing fine. Doesn't associate with other patients. Cooperative."

"Skin lesions appear on patient's legs."

"Sometimes sits in Day Room and colors." "This patient is walking around with crayons in her hand." "Has abrasion on chin and cut on lips. When asked what happened, said she tripped and fell."

"Fell on the driveway. Shoes have a run down appearance. Right leg appears to be turned in. Took hold of my arm to walk with (something she will hardly ever do)."

"Easter basket was bought out of patient's funds and put on her bed. Look what Easter bunny brought you, Regina, I said. Was real delighted and nurse asked her if rabbit came through the window and she said, 'Well that's nice.'"

"From time to time we have to give her Sodium Amytal to quiet her down if she gets out of bounce [sic]."

"Patient is receiving Aquafor for rash, Mellaril, 200 mg. q.i.d., Stelazine, 20 mg. b.i.d., Thorazine, 400 mg. q.i.d., and Artane, 2 mg. liquid daily."

REGINA'S RECORD

"Regina is a girl who is completely disoriented, deteriorated. All functions are nil."

"Vomited mucus after her meds were given. Gagging this p.m."

"Her legs seem to buckle. Complaining of pain in both hips." "Often states: It's all right, I want to die soon anyway." "Continues to walk with a limp. Knees on left leg red and raw."

"Stomach cramps. Has diarrhea. Bed and pajamas were soiled."

"Regina is unable to reach second step when coming in back door. Patient used great effort and could not make it without help."

"Birthday card received from her mother. Regina is 53 today."

October 10, 1974

"Patient is an old deteriorating schizophrenic. She is a loner on the ward, does not communicate with others, weak legs, needs help dressing herself and with other minor chores."

D. Obreccase, MD
October 14, 1974

"Patient fell while on the way to OT while walking over painter's drop cloth. Struck nose on floor. Moderate amount of bleeding noted. Nose still swollen from previous fall."

"Returning from walk with group, patient starting listing to the right and fell on her face while she was walking down the sidewalk. Abrasion on right cheek bone. Patient has bruise under left eye from previous fall." *"Patient fell out on the porch, then fell again on chair in Day Room landing on both knees. Appears unable to see. Request eye examination."*

"Patient came off elevator through the door into AB hallway, bumped into another patient and, to avoid bumping into laundry cart, fell hitting nose. Has scrape on nose."

"Regina fell by her own bed on two occasions this a.m. Left knee bruised."

"Patient ran into door and fell on floor hitting forehead. Immediately forehead started to swell. Had a swelling about one and one half inches in diameter. Patient unresponsive, pale and fainted." *"Patient struck head again this a.m. Slight swelling behind right ear. Stated, 'I'm okay.'"*

REGINA'S RECORD

> *"Regina is crying again this afternoon. She says she wants to die soon and she can't. Check meds."*

In 1979, 13,409 psychiatric patients were on anti-psychotic medications, 86.8 percent were taking one major tranquilizer, 12.5 percent were taking two, and 0.7 percent were taking three. Regina was prescribed four and five on a regular basis. By the end of 1979, she had swallowed over 97,500 pills.

"Miss Van Amber is: Schizophrenic, disorganized type. Paranoid schizophrenic. Paranoid. Schizophrenic, unclassified. Catatonic. Schizophrenic with autistic references. Autistic. A severely regressed schizophrenic. Schizophrenic – flat affective type. Confused schizophrenic with salad-type language. Incompetent. Violent at times. Uncooperative. Aggressive. Anxious. Passive. An old burnt out schizophrenic. Someone who can never live on the outside. Schizoaffective type. Chronic undifferentiated type. Mute. Weak. Very strong. Someone who sees herself as an ugly duckling. A loner. Fearful. Deteriorating. Unkempt. Clean. Someone with a high opinion of herself. Unemployable. Smoking risk. Delusional. Bizarre behaviors. Negativistic. Paranoid. Not addicted to drugs. A threat to herself and others. Congenial. Not insane. Deep in thought. Cooperative. Uncooperative. Uncomfortable in either sexual role. Afraid of men. . . . an old lady! . . . a girl. Afraid of aides. [a] Patient. Beneficiary. Subject. Queen. Mrs. Miss. Ms. Regina. Patient Van Amber. Classic case of schizophrenia, hebephrenic type. Hallucinatory. Someone with almost no insight. Below average IQ. Higher than average IQ. Above average intelligence. Immature. Intelligent. Has had one abortion. Has had several children. Extremely ill. Sick. Myopic. Has had sex with several men. Elated. Depressed. Not depressed. Sad. Crying."

"Regina can't hardly see at all. Doesn't she wear glasses?"

"There is no place for her here. This is the worst case of schizophrenia I ever saw."
L. McManus, MD
April, 1975

"Could funds be taken from her account? Regina likes to read Wisconsin Magazine and would like a year's subscription."

"Regina is such a sad little soul who stays off by herself curled in a chair."

"Please do not put throw rugs near Miss Van Amber's bed. She has slipped on them in the past."

"Please do not put throw rugs near Patient Van Amber's chair. She slipped and fell last week while getting up for meal time."

REGINA'S RECORD

"Please ask janitorial staff not to put rugs near Regina's bed."

"Miss Van Amber fell in the Day Room this p.m. and struck her head on the floor.

"She could not get up on her own. Taken to bed with help of aides."

"Regina is crying this a.m. Unable to get out of bed."

"O Little Town of Bethlehem"

Theresa Udelhofen, Grandma's youngest sister, believed what a lot of others believe about miracles and spiritual visitations. Theresa was so rigorously dedicated to daily rituals in the Catholic faith, the Good Sisters of Notre Dame in Mankato, Minnesota, allowed her the right to move into their four-story convent, live out her holy existence with them. And she did.

Theresa was a short, stocky woman with a large face and tight facial skin seemingly forced that way by the power of her hair bun. Those who viewed her external life around the convent and during mass, saw someone of conviction and prayer, but rituals are deceiving and inside the convent's subdued walls, inside the quiet rooms and dim hallways, Theresa often whispered private contempt for her three older sisters and their families. She felt that lack of faith had brought them misery and suffering which would come to an end if only they would repent.

In the early Seventies, after Regina's transfer to Tomah, Theresa learned of the "miracle" images of Jesus seen in a tree near Nacedah, Wisconsin, a few hours' drive across the border from Mankato. She made a pilgrimage to the site, bought religious symbols and cards for relatives, shared her insights with the good sisters, and each time placed herself a notch or two higher on the ladder toward heaven's acceptance.

Her pilgrimage became a yearly event.

Many shared Theresa's belief about the tree in Nacedah. Thousands visited, saw what they wanted to see, hoped the place would soon become officially sanctified by the Catholic Church as a holy shrine.

Patricia Gertasen, the head nurse in the women's section at Tomah VA, was also a true believer. The two met for the first time during a visit Theresa had made to the ward in 1974. Theresa demanded that Regina go to confession and attend Mass on a regular basis, that a priest be involved in her treatment, and that power of attorney over Regina's affairs be given to her. She told Gertasen that the reasons for her requests were sound because her oldest sister (my grandmother) was insane, and Regina's brothers and sisters didn't care.

Gertasen was deeply moved by Theresa's concern, went to work to implement what my great aunt had requested. She asked the weekend shift to escort Regina to Saturday evening confessions and Sunday Mass, asked the regular staff to escort Regina to all Holy Days of Obligation, and made inquiries into Theresa's request for power of attorney (Mother's oldest brother Marvin had power of attorney).

Gertasen, who referred to patients in the female section as "my girls" contacted a local priest who agreed to sit in on weekly "team therapy" sessions with Regina.

Regina suffered at least two injuries going to and from Catholic services yet, each year Theresa visited, the first question she asked the Tomah staff was whether or not Regina was going to confession, attending Mass, and seeing a priest in therapy.

On her last recorded visit, Theresa tracked down Gertasen, said she had been to the "Jesus tree" in Nacedah, told the nurse that my grandmother was dead and that I had turned out be a "very nice young man who owned a large cattle farm in Alaska".

Gertasen wrote down every word.

>"For her noon meal today she ate a salad, mashed potatoes and gravy, diced carrots and ham. Her manners are good. Her hair is combed, her lipstick and fingernail polish appear neat, but her dress is unbuttoned. I asked to join her and she said it was okay and seemed pleased when I did. I asked Regina what she remembered about her past and she said that, a long time ago, she watched an eclipse of the sun. I asked her what she remembered about it and she stated that it was none of my business. 'You can't know what I've seen. Isn't that enough?'"

September 25, 1975 Ward Report, Tomah VA
    Problem #1. Schizophrenia, hebephrenic type.
    Problem #2. Obesity. Present weight is 141.
    Problem #3. Psoriasis, fungus infection of the toes.
    Problem #4. Borderline EKG.
    Problem #5. Placement. This is constantly being worked on by the Social Worker.
    Problem #6. Fracture of nasal bone without displacement, resolved.
    Problem #7. Contact dermatitis, resolved.
    Problem #8. Peripheral abscess with fistula of rectum.
    Problem #9. Fracture of right large toe, resolved.
    Problem #10. Rash on face, resolved.
    Problem #11. Severe trichomonas, resolved.
    Problem #12. Tumor, left, lateral aspect, left leg, biopsy done, resolved. No malignancy.

> *Problem #13, 14, and 15. Deleted.*
> *Problem #16. Chronic constipation. No medication.*
> *Problem #17. Longitudinal lordosis due to muscle spasm, no treatment at present time."*

On December 25th, 1978, during Christmas service in the chapel, my mother, tormented by ongoing side effects from multiple doses of psychotropic pills, limping from a swollen right ankle caused by another fall and unable to see well (with or without glasses), interrupted the Mass with a song. The aides moved through the pews to quiet her down, but the priest, apparently struck by the moment, turned, said it was okay to let her continue.

Regina sang "O Little Town of Bethlehem" in that odd squeak of a voice, and after Mass the priest met her at the door, thanked her, wished her a Merry Christmas.

She stopped, raised her head, and, according to the report, "for the first time in many months [she] grinned and said, '*And a Merry Christmas to you, priest.*'"

In April of 1979, as her falling continued, one nurse wrote that she was given "open ward privileges" allowed to go to the canteen unescorted, and free (with permission) to walk by herself around the hospital grounds. She only went out once in late spring, limped across the parking lot to a grassy area, came back after a few minutes, told Nurse Gallison that she saw dandelions everywhere. "And are they ever nice," she said.

Her crayon artwork won first prize in a ward contest in July, and that same month she was assigned a female physician for the first time.

The Blue Cart

On January 13, 1983, at around ten o'clock in the evening, Regina fell again in the Day Room. She tried getting up, attempted to push herself off the floor and rise, as she had risen so many times before. Not this time.

The aides lifted her into a wheelchair, escorted her to bed. The following morning she told aides that she couldn't get out of bed, and as they attempted to lift her, she let out a cry, held her side and said, "My hip!" After some discussion they wheeled her to X-ray, learned her hip was broken and called for a car to drive her down the interstate to the Madison VA Medical Center.

The intake nurse in Madison wrote her age as 60 (she was 61) and added that Regina had been "a psychiatric patient for 11 years".

Surgery was scheduled for early the following morning. There was no room available on the all-male ward in orthopedics so they moved her bed into a small waiting area near the nurses' station, and drew up two divider curtains for privacy.

The early morning operation had gone well, according to the surgeon, and his team moved her into the recovery room where she would awaken in a few minutes from her deep sleep state.

One of the rooms in Orthopedics had opened up and the staff pushed her bed there for more privacy.

Most of the day she was in and out of sleep, struggled

REGINA'S RECORD

somewhat against the IVs and attempted once to pull them out. The staff put restraints on her wrists, checked on her during rounds, took her blood pressure, and noted that everything was normal.

Light snow was gently falling outside her window.

The night nurse made her rounds about 12:20 a.m., saw that Regina was awake, asked her how she was feeling.

"I'm not answering any more questions," she said. "It's none of your business. Get out."

1:40 a.m

"Is this Mr. Marvin Van Amber?"

"Yes."

"Mr. Van Amber, this is Betty Lern, the Administrative Officer at the VA Hospital in Madison, Wisconsin calling."

"Yes."

"And Doctor Mayes is on the other phone here and would like to talk to you about your sister Regina. Now do we have your permission to record this conversation for her record? It would just be a part of her record."

"Oh, OK."

"OK, here is Dr. Mayes and then when he is finished there are some other things I would like to talk to you about."

"Hello Mr. Van Amber, this is Dr. Mayes. I am on-call at the VA Hospital tonight. I am calling you for Dr. Bagge who is the Orthopedic Resident taking care of your sister. She passed away tonight I am afraid to say. We are not really sure what exactly happened. She may have swallowed something and had it go down the wrong way so to speak – in the windpipe and had stopped breathing. And we resuscitated her and tried to bring her around for quite some time and there were quite a few of us in there working with her but we were just unable to do so."

"So I just needed to call you and let you know about what has happened here tonight. Now is there any possibility – I have talked with Dr. Bagge who is not in the hospital right now – but we were both wondering if there would be any way you, as her next of kin, would consent to allowing us to take a look at things, to perform an autopsy on Regina. And just try to get to the bottom of what actually happened tonight. Would you think that would be a reasonable thing to do?"

"I guess it would probably be all right."

"I hate to ask and press for something like this so soon after you have heard about her, but I think it would be helpful for us here and it might also help you folks in terms of knowing exactly what happened. And I think it would be beneficial for both of us if that would be OK with you?"

"I guess it would."

"OK, all right sir."

"Where will she be buried? Will the VA take care of it?"

"How about if I have you talk with the Medical Administrator here after I get off the line and you can discuss those things with her. Is that OK?"

"OK."

"OK, do you have any other questions that I could answer?"

"Well, I can hardly think right now."

"Yes, OK, well, I am very, very sorry and we will let you talk with the Medical Administrator here and ask her some of those types of questions about what will happen from here."

"OK, this is Betty Lern again, do you know the name of the funeral home that you will be making arrangements with?"

"Well, do you think she will be shipped back here?"

"Well, that is whatever you want – whatever your plans are."

"Well, I just don't know what to say."

"Unless you wanted to think about it and get back to us."

"Well, why not do that. Do you have a number I can call back?"

"Sure."

End of transcription.

Uncle Marvin's presence was more of a surprise to me than the blast of January cold that morning. It was just after seven, and I wasn't fully awake, drummed out of a dream when the knocking began. But even in my daze I noticed something odd about the way Marvin was dressed, not his nylon parka or dark slacks or leather boots, but something else I wasn't sure about until after he began the conversation. Whatever the reason for his presence I was certain it was going to be brief because the hum of his Ford pickup idling near the curb behind him suggested he was there to leave quickly. What was different about him, I suddenly realized, was the absence of anything on his head. His caps more than his cars or pickups revealed changes in his life. Once advertising seed or feed or herbicide or tractor companies, caps with faded bills, torn, dirty – those caps had been replaced by Arctic Cat or Polaris or some fishing reel outfit. But new or old, what they all had in common was that none of his caps sat on his head any other way but tilted as if things mattered more at an angle. But this morning, in the doorway, whatever had been on his head was out of sight, and made him appear both fragile and reverent.

He didn't come in. He held the outside door open with one elbow, his hands hidden inside his coat pockets, a soft wooden glaze in his eyes, sad, as he worked out his words careful and slow, tagged heavy with the frozen breath of morning whiskey.

"Say," he began slowly, "I got a bad call from the Veterans' people last night, Jimmy. Regina died around one o'clock. She swallowed something wrong I guess and her heart couldn't take it is pretty much what they said."

I looked away, muttered something about people in institutions living a long time.

"God, I thought that she would, too."

Marvin showed no emotion, avoided any direct glance, offered nothing further but an awkward silence until he finally mumbled that he had better get over to the nursing home and tell Grandma, then, after another long pause – a man not certain where to look, what to do, what more could be said – he turned to leave, hesitated. "We was there a couple of years ago," he said. "Christmas." He slipped a photograph from his pocket, handed it to me. "You can have that," he said. And in a quiet tone delivered by this untrained messenger of death, he rubbed the side of his face, stared at his boots as if they held a reminder of something curious, and said, "I'm awfully sorry, Jimmy."

By the time my thoughts cleared long enough to engage him with more questions, Marvin was on his way to the pickup. I'm not sure why I didn't call him back, ask him why he waited so God damn long to tell me about Mother's death. Fear mixed with respect maybe, and the idea I'd had for a long time that in some manipulated future situation there would be a way to craft Marvin into a neutral place, take the risk and seduce him to let go of his secrets, ask why he slapped Regina in his kitchen way back when. But that didn't happen and maybe because there are no perfect settings to discuss madness, or rage – or maybe because I was never quite certain that Marvin wouldn't go berserk and punch me in the face, or maybe because all of us had practised omission so long that nothing much mattered when it came to Regina.

I looked at the photo. It revealed a woman hunched into a defensive posture, someone who appeared frozen in a permanent shiver from a steady draught, a woman seemingly fearful of an imminent beating, someone staring reluctantly through loose features with ancient, leery eyes like a medieval child who had squinted one side of her face into a wary expression, uncertain what horrid pain the camera or its holder might bring.

I looked at that picture for a long time, went into the bedroom and told my wife about Regina.

"My mother is dead."

It seemed like such and odd thing to say. Strange to use 'my' and 'mother' in the same sentence.

After the Blue Cart emergency team was called, the last needle in Regina's faded existence came slamming through her breastplate, driven with terrific force into her quiet heart. The adrenaline did nothing, the OD set the time of death, and aides wheeled her to the morgue where a pathologist sawed open her chest, took out her heart, weighed it, took out everything else, looked, checked her lungs, wrote down "pulmonary edema" as cause of death, sawed open her skull, pulled her flesh mask down off her face, severed the brain stem, prised out her brain, weighed it, then put it in a jar for later research study at the university. He poured plaster of Paris into her skull, pulled up her facemask, stapled things together, and went for coffee.

Mother's body came back to Alexandria without clothes. The funeral director called me, said they had an extra dress they could put on her, if I wanted, and a beautician would stop over and fix her hair.

The VA paid for her casket and I picked out the memorial card from a tray of four selections. The announcement in the paper said that Mother had been gone many years, that she had once worked near Chicago and later in Wisconsin. The local announcer on the Silvertone repeated the obituary on the air.

My good wife and family, I am still ashamed to say, had never met my mother, and after the body was ready for viewing we walked the few blocks across Broadway to the funeral home. I went ahead a little, guessing which of two rooms she was in. I excused myself in the first one when I saw Tom Anderson, the young funeral director, near a dark haired woman so perfect in her casket. He acted surprised when I asked where my mother was.

"This is the right room," he answered.

The woman in the picture my Uncle Marvin had handed me a day earlier was not the same person as the woman in the casket. Except for a large bruise on the right side of her head behind the hairline, her face had no contorted features, no ancient glaze, no drug induced twisted expressions, anything that would indicate a lifetime existence inside a mental hospital.

"This is my mother, Regina," I said to my family, and apologized again for not taking them to see her. "This is her."

During the evening prayer service the priest suffered a sudden attack of diarrhea and had to leave. Family members reciting the Rosary lost track. The singer and organist got their times mixed up, arrived after the service was over.

Grandma died four weeks later. She struggled for three days at the end, passed away in the morning surrounded by family. I had kissed her lips, said good-bye the night before and there is no reason to doubt that here was a good person on this earth, filled with a peace at last that her youngest daughter had finally come home.

One year earlier, for the first time in her life, Grandma was forced to receive welfare after she could no longer walk and had to be admitted to a nursing home. The cost for a single room with minimum care had jumped far beyond her ability to pay. Six months after she had been admitted, she quietly complained (which was rare) that early one morning an aide responsible for helping her out of bed had shoved her hard into her wheelchair then angrily maneuvered her sore legs and feet into place in a thoughtless, uncaring way. My grandmother was frightened. I was furious, wrote a stern letter of protest to the home's administration, got an answer that there had "never been a history of abuse in the home" and the incident had not happened. I met with the chief administrator following her written response and she once again assured me that "nothing had happened".

Before my grandmother's body was removed from her room in the nursing home, Aunt Digna showed up, upset everyone by boxing up her things, telling everyone they could come out later to her home to pick through what was left.

A week after Mother died I wrote to the VA in Tomah and Downey VA in North Chicago. I thanked them for their years of service to my mother, asked the people in Tomah about a large bruise on her head. A month passed, then two, and when there was no response, no acknowledgement of anything. I wondered about that large wound and what it meant. Around that same time I began to have recurring nightmares about Regina, variations of someone laughing in a hysterical way before pushing her down a flight of steps. I am at the bottom with no arms.

Noreen Van Amber Stewart, Mother's second oldest sister, rose before her husband one morning. She went directly to the medicine cabinet, took out a bottle of pills, walked down in the basement near the old cistern where some of us kids had written our names with flaming Farmer matches on the low ceiling.

The farm was quiet. Cows were in the pasture. The dog was

asleep under the granary. The garden was heavy with dew.

Noreen tied a clothesline around her neck, knotted it tight over a rafter, gulped the bottle of pills, dropped her arms, then fell backwards as she thrust her legs out. The cord stretched. Her head came to rest two inches from the floor. Her eyes were fixed on the cobwebs, her mouth open with pills not yet swallowed, her good husband then rising, wondering, looking, calling her name, wondering, seeing the pale of her legs, rushing down the basement steps, calling her to rise again, holding her precious neck, pleading through the last sounds of calling out her name in the belly of their home.

Noreen had been to see Regina the year before. She asked the nurses why her sister was drooling and staring off into space, why her head was moving this way and that, twitching, jerking, jerky spasms. Why are her hands trembling like that, she asked.

When she got back to the farm, she wrote the VA a four-page letter of protest; a go to hell letter that didn't go far enough, but the only family letter saved in the records. "You people can do much better with my sister, Regina. Why do you have to keep her so drugged up with pills? I know a lot about pills," she said. "I've suffered, too."

Her husband told her that the effort was useless. "Do you think the VA is going to listen to you?"

"Well, at least I did something," she said. "At least I tried."

A few years earlier Noreen's youngest daughter, Carol, was hitchhiking back from a college dance in South Carolina with her boyfriend. A pickup truck slowed, stopped, and Carol opened the door, greeted the driver, and started to get in with her boyfriend close behind. The driver grabbed Carol's arm before she could retreat, sped off with tires spitting gravel. Carol fought her attacker while her boyfriend stood helpless back on the road. Carol screamed, got loose long enough to throw herself out of the speeding truck, but the man caught her by the ankle and would not let go, dragging her on the road, her head bouncing on the pavement. By the time she was able to get free she was almost dead.

It took her two years to recover, but she has no sense of smell.

Noreen's middle daughter, Laura, had just returned home from work to her Minneapolis apartment and was changing clothes in her bedroom when a stranger slid out from under her bed and attacked. Laura got hold of his left hand, sunk her teeth into his right index finger, and bit it completely off. A neighbor heard his screams and called police as the man escaped. Police followed the blood trail to a nearby apartment complex where they arrested the attacker.

In mid-summer, 1991, Marvin, Regina's oldest brother, got a call from his youngest daughter Lucy. The call woke him. It was well after midnight. His wife Digna got up at almost the same time. Something was wrong. Lucy told her father that Missy, her oldest daughter, was missing. Missy was attending St. Cloud State University and three days from graduating with an elementary education degree. After working the late shift at a resort complex in Alexandria, Missy drove the sixty miles to her apartment in St. Cloud. She greeted her roommate who was up late studying for finals. She told her roommate that she was going to take one of their new puppies for a fifteen-minute walk. It was just after midnight, three blocks from campus. The night was hot.

Was she naive? the police asked. Was she responsible? Did she have a boyfriend? Where was he now? Could she have decided to hit the bars before closing? Was she a dressed in a certain specific way? What exactly was she wearing? Was she someone who would go wild at night and not come back for a few days? What about the puppy?

Three days later, following a useless search and posters everywhere, police questioned a handsome young rapist who had just been released from a nearby prison. They determined that he had not been picked up by the state parole bus that was supposed to take him to his half way house in Minneapolis, discovered he simply walked away without further supervision to watch a Fourth of July parade before stealing a Camaro, a knife, a gun, rope – waited in the car near the college for a woman, any woman, and then Missy came walking through the dark.

He got out of the car as she strolled past, moved quickly and carefully behind her, Say Miss, asked where such and such was, then stuck the gun in her neck, grabbed her arm, pulled her into the car, threw her dog in the back seat, told her to lay on the floor, to say nothing, tied her wrists to the brake pedal, stepped on her throat with his left foot, and told her that if she moved he would kill the puppy. He drove out to the country, found a wood, dragged her from the car, dragged her pleading Why are you doing this? Down through a ditch, pulled her begging Please don't hurt me into the tree line, ripped off her clothes, raped her, slashed her throat as she prayed to Jesus, weeping. He cut the puppy's throat, went back to the car, drove to a nearby town, ate scrambled eggs, toast and bacon, dabbed the corner of his mouth with the complimentary napkin, tipped the waitress, drove to his mother's house to rest, have a few beers, smoke, knowing that, if he were ever caught, they would only send him back to where he came from and nothing bad would happen.

The state of Minnesota, of course, assumed no culpability.

REGINA'S RECORD

By 1995, at least 18 females in my grandparents' direct and extended family of 33, one way or another, one after another, in the country and in the city, walking on a road, riding on a train, in a hospital, at home, in a nursing home, in a car – mothers, sisters, wives, aunts, daughters, granddaughters, cousins, second cousins – had been assaulted. Skull fractures, rape, attempted rape, burns, bruises, beatings, broken bones, suicide, sexual abuse, horrified as children, murdered in cold blood.

There is nothing civilized about life in America. We are the most violent society on earth. And we rarely listen to what the dead are trying to tell us.

"I had the most wonderful time."

Letters and postcards 1943 to 1945

I'm working at Sacred Heart (Spokane, Washington) now. I don't know why I get so tired, but sometimes I feel like I could sleep for a week.

I stayed awake half the night listening to voices from the next room. They were having a party and talking loudly and the cussing was terrible. They were drunk and mad at the Japanese. One man kept saying he was going to kill as many Japs as he could. Maybe on Saturday I'll get a chance to sleep in.

I try to make daily mass at the hospital. The priest is nice. I think I'll skip tomorrow, I'm exhausted.

Betty and I went to a show starring Bob Hope and Bing Crosby. It was a lot of fun and how we laughed. Tomorrow I'm going to talk to the recruiter again and try to join up.

They accepted me in the WACs. I leave for basic in two weeks. I'm so happy.

Des Moines isn't a bad place. I went on sick call today with a chest cold. I should get my orders soon. Hopefully it will be England. I've always wanted to go there.

Well, I can't believe I'm in San Francisco. It's such a beautiful city, and Market Street must be the busiest place on earth.

REGINA'S RECORD

When I heard over the radio that President Roosevelt had just died I was very sad. I told the First Sergeant and he said, Kathy, you shouldn't say things like that when it's not true.

I twisted my ankle in softball practice and couldn't play on Sunday. We're still in first place. Guess I'll have to sit on the bench and cheer them on. I hope we win.

They started painting the office yesterday and the paint made me nauseous. I didn't eat supper, and went to bed early. Today I still feel awful.

That paint I told you about really made me sick. I was in my room for two days just exhausted and throwing up. Hope to feel better by Monday. We have Post inspection at 0930.

Gosh, I almost ran over the Post Chaplain with my bicycle. I wasn't watching where I was going and narrowly avoided hitting him. How embarrassing! Well, another month and I'll be caught up with Sis (Noreen) in rank.

How is everything at Fort Dix? I put in for overseas duty. I hope I get England. Betty and I went into San Francisco last week. We met a man on Market Street who invited us to hear a speaker talk about the poor of the world. When we went inside the people were very nice and welcomed us. I signed up to attend another meeting in the Fall. By the way, I haven't forgotten about the five dollars you loaned me. Payday is tomorrow, and I'll be sure to send it along.

Betty and I went into Santa Rosa for the weekend. There is a little park there with the most beautiful flower garden.

I know by now that you've heard the news about VJ day. Well, Betty and I went into San Francisco and people were everywhere celebrating and dancing in the streets. I was so glad to be there. I've never seen anything like it. Everyone was so happy. I had the most wonderful time.

Please don't worry about me. I'll be getting my discharge as soon as they release me from the hospital. I don't know what will happen after that. Maybe I'll die. Sorry to be so gloomy. I've just had the blues lately.

Well, it's over. I'm writing this on the train and I'll mail it when we get to Portland. I'll switch there and catch the first train to Spokane. After I rest for a few days, I'll look for work and then come home when I get the first chance. It will be good to see everyone. I'm sure we'll all have a lot of catching up to do. I love you, Mama. Kiss Papa for me.

Love, Reggie

Love, Regina

All my love, Regina

Love, Sis

REGINA'S RECORD

PS. The weather was perfect.
>Kiss the kids for me. They're so sweet and I miss them. It will be good to come home again. Soon as I can.

Dear Jimmy and Mary,

I wanted to be sure and tell you that old Ted died on Wednesday. The County nurse found his body. She used to check on him once a month, I guess, because she was worried that if his older brother, Louie, went out there and found him dead, Louie would bury him in the garden.

It got me to thinking about some of the times when you were growing up. I'm glad you were with me all those years. It wasn't always easy for us but I'm sure you know that I did the best I could. I pray for you and your family every night, Jimmy. You're lucky to have such a wonderful wife and those boys are so sweet and good, and I miss them a lot. I hope you can come for Easter if the weather is nice.

Love, Gramma

PS Do you want that old radio? Why don't you take it with you the next time you come. It still works real good.

>*"There is a picture of a young man and his family on her wall and it was upside down. It this a relative?"*
>
> Ann Parks, RN

"Do I know you from somewhere?"

There is a fight in The Pink Pussy Cat Lounge around ten o'clock, and I'm clubbed on the side of my face by someone, falling to the floor with the bark of dogs.
    There is a fight in the parking lot outside the Brass Rail at around eleven and I'm on the pavement trying to understand the dull of flashing lights.
    There is a fight in the doorway to Fargo's Fabulous Five Spot. I'm on the sidewalk. I taste salt from blood running out of my nose.
    A shoving match outside the Holiday Inn bar near midnight means something, but I'm not sure what.
    Repeated fists to the face from one of two in the front seat to one in the back seat inside a squad car after midnight.
    I remember clearly the cop's words, "If I ever . . ."
    There is blood and vomit near the curb in the dark parking lot outside Red Owl Foods.
    There is the sound of continuous hacking and vomiting inside the men's can in Pa Dogg's All Night Pizza.
    There is the loud rumble from a blue Ford Galaxy 500 moving down the on-ramp on I-94 east toward Fergus Falls, Minnesota. The Galaxy's right windshield wiper has scratched a half moon in the glass, but it's nothing compared to the driver's side where a rock spit from a truck tire imprinted a large butterfly. There is a hole in the muffler and part of the tail pipe is missing.
    There is the sound of coughing and running water inside the rest room at the Fergus Falls Texaco Station. My driver's

license expired a year ago. Tabs on the license plates are six months overdue. I should call my wife.

State hospital Next Right. Regina is there. The right front headlight doesn't work on low beam. People get pissed when you're driving with brights. The driver's side window crank is sheered off, broken.

There is the sound of coughing and running water inside the rest room at a truck stop near Alexandria, Minnesota. Grandma is sleeping behind the green divider, surrounded by old boxes and dust, sleeping near a small nightstand that I made for her in shop class. Doctors say she has an enlarged heart.

There is the continuous rumble from the Ford Galaxy past the St. Cloud, Minnesota exit sign. St. Cloud Veterans' Administration Hospital, Next Right. Who decides about these signs and where to put them? Who?

There is an announcement on the Ford's radio that the Reverend Billy Graham has promised a Crusade for Christ in Minneapolis. Everyone will be welcome. Admission free. I should go. Something might happen. I could walk down and gather with the others when the calls goes out, get a close look at Billy.

The passenger side mirror is cracked. St. Anthony of Padua, Finder of Lost Things is on the dashboard. He is missing a hand.

There is the sound of running water inside the rest room at the Trucker's Plaza in St. Paul – the rumbling racket from the Ford Galaxy heading east southeast toward the Wisconsin border.

Welcome to Wisconsin.

Menomonie Next Right.

Eau Claire Next Right. The great Henry Aaron played in Eau Claire.

Tomah Next Right.

Tomah VA Next Right.

It has been raining for two hundred God damn miles.

I don't know why I'm here. I'll tell them I'm here to see my mother. I'll raise my voice a little, but not too much. No one will question me. Why would they question me? I really should have a date handy in case someone asks. "Yes, it's September, 1973." Tenth? Eleventh? Who cares? No one will ask. If they do I'll tell them to go look it up. "Look it up," I'll say. "I'm here to visit someone."

Low thunder. I hate mornings. Mornings are depressing enough when it's not raining. My cheek is swollen, sore to the touch where the cop smacked me. My jaw pops when I try to open wide.

I've got to do something about crap on the floor – candy wrappers, beer cans, faded parking tickets, hardened gum lining the ashtray, a used food stamp booklet, dirt and grime everywhere. I've got to clean up this mess, sometime.

It continues to rain – pelting the car with drops larger now than before. Thunder cracks over the car's rumble. The radio leaps to static then silence. I pound the dash with a fist. That's what you do when it doesn't work. Pound the fucking dash. Hammer a fist hard down on it again and again and again until St. Anthony is bouncing, dust rising – pound it until it's right and it works and everything is clear without static again.

I turn off the engine and decide to make a run for the nearest building. My legs hurt. My face hurts. My body aches. I should have bought a razor, shaved when I was dowsing my face with the shock of water back at the truck stop between gagging and puking and coughing. I'm not that dirty. I tug down my baseball cap, nudge the car door open to a rusty screech that always hurts my teeth, then run, puddle jumping all the way to those first steps, take three at a time up, and I'm inside looking down this one long hallway that must end somewhere, but where?

Might be too early. Or too late. I'll walk and look. I won't ask anyone about anything until I absolutely have to. I won't look down or up. Look straight ahead, eyes fixed on a distant point like I know exactly what I want, what I'm doing, where I'm going. But not too fixed. No thousand yard stare. People notice.

"Excuse me. I'm here to see Regina Van Amber," I say to the woman leaning over a table in OT.

The woman turns a little, peers over the top of her glasses, slips a fistful of leather punches back in their slot-tray on the table, speaks without looking up. "Regina's not here today," she says sternly. "I'll have to go get her."

It has been difficult for me to swallow. The right side of my neck is swollen, but I'm not sure how it got that way.

Regina stands now at the top of the second floor stairs. Her left hand trembles on the rail as she descends almost sideways, head down, eyes on her difficult purpose. The OT woman is beside her, a bit ahead of her and down one step, then another, guiding yet not touching her, one finger pointing out where to step and she's saying, "That's right. That's good."

Yellow chain links guard the center of the stairwell. A waist high strip a few inches wide is worn to bare metal from fingers that have grazed it, clutched it for moments.

Regina has not seen me yet, still watching her feet, watching as her faded blue slippers move down one more step and the last, bounces a little on floor level, her head in slight motion, her short hair glazed white over her ears, choppy. She's a little cutie pie. She's a real sweetie all right. And one nice print dress, white sweater with a few splotches of something or other that doesn't matter. A little munchkin I say she is, a tiny woman really, a small woman, a woman shrunken and frail with age well beyond what she is – old and small now, much older than the last time I saw her when she left the room and I couldn't see straight through my own tears, my endless uncontrolled sobbing, until I could have a drink.

My mind fills with sudden questions. Should I do this this way with my hands or that way with my hands? What do people do on these occasions, anyway? My hands out of my pockets, hands behind my back, in front folded over my belt buckle, stupid hands, could hug her. Be careful here. What might possibly be appropriate for this important occasion? Oh, she seems wounded, afraid maybe. And I just don't know what to do with my fucking hands, drop them down, so I drop them down, realizing after a thought or two that – Jesus, are you kidding me? I'm standing at full attention, rigid and right out of a manual for royalty.

"Who could it be?" she says smiling like kid-happy, no, half her face is smiling, without looking up she's smiling, lips cracked and dry she's smiling, cheekbones puffed, puffier on one side, flared, swollen. Christ, we match. But I am too far away. She shuffles closer, little shuffle slides, baby steps, her head in motion with that slight shake every now and then – green eyes of a child. Hey, how are you, Mister Fantastic? What blew you into town? Does your face give it away? Examine, please, a Picasso, some incredible drawing he did at nineteen; some small perfect sketch on a note pad, smaller than usual, needs closer attention to detail. A foot away, three inches, and I'm not moving, not exhaling until she draws back. And when she does, I breathe and say to myself: Jesus God, this is your mother, man. I am her son.

"I don't know," she says. "Do you work here? Do I know you from somewhere?"

"I'm Jimmy," I say. "Came to visit. Would you like coffee?

Or a soda maybe. We could try the canteen – if it's all right."
"Yes," she said. "The canteen."
"I'll go then," her escort says. "You go ahead."
"Do I know you?"
"I'm your son, James – Jimmy." That's louder than I wanted. "Do you remember me?"
"No," she says. "I don't remember you."
"Do you remember Gramma?"
"Gramma? No. No, I don't remember Gramma."
"You're a grandmother now too, you know," I say. "Boys. Grandsons."
"Sons. Sons are good. I like sons."

The canteen is perfect. Other patients in line, and someone in long white breezes past in a mad blur, reaches between patients for what he wants, nudges one human being to step aside without excuse me, sir, reaches in front of another human being as if the man could not exist, didn't suffer enough for his sins, then goes to the head of the line, pays the cashier, leaves. I want to rush after him, say just a minute you asshole, but I don't. I'm with Mother as she reaches into her sweater pocket, fumbles with a coupon booklet, trying now to tear one from the staple, her little finger out of control, hooking wildly, her thumb and finger unable to free the coupon, her hands active, jerking out of control. Oh, and her right shoulder is the shoulder I touch, shake my head, but not too much, nothing to alarm her, startle her tender soul.

"Let me."

The table is perfect. Mother sips her soda, looks to me, my face, examining, grinning, not blinking, now blinking, not grinning, examining. I'm grinning then not grinning, blinking too. We're blinking. Not grinning. Now we're grinning. Now we're grinning and blinking and sipping from our straws like friends, lovers, nutty kids at a drugstore fountain sipping from our striped straws, grinning.

"Did you bump something?"

"No," I say. "Not really. I'm okay. It's nothing."

"I have to go now," she says with panic in her voice.

"Couldn't you . . . maybe a little longer? Stay a while longer, please. I mean, wouldn't that be all right?"

"Yes, I suppose, but I still have to go. You have to go, too," she says. "Don't you? You'll want to get back there."

"Yes, I suppose."

"Yes," she says.

"Yes."

"Okay, then. Will we do this again?"

"Yes," she says. "What will we do?"

"Okay. Well, You know. Whatever."

"Would it be okay, you know, maybe I could kiss you when you leave. Not if it hurts or anything – I wouldn't want anything you wouldn't want, you know. Nothing like that."

"Yes. Yes. You could kiss me. Did you kiss me before?"

"A while ago?"

"Yes, before – a while ago."

"Sure," I say. "Of course. Oh yes. Do you remember that?"

"No. Who are you? I can't figure you out."

"It's all right."

We are leaving, moving through the hallway, walking close, an inch from touching arms and shoulders, looking once through the windows at pouring rain, sheets, rice-like, swept in swirls by the wind. We have the hallway to ourselves this day, walking to its end until we are standing where we met and she turns, raising her arm, her right hand to touch the left side of my burning face, her one finger extended, wiggle-wagging, wanting I'm sure to heal the swelling on my cheek with her tenderness, wanting to stop the throb, but instead she flinches, sees a flaw in her method, retreats a step, moves close again, twists her neck, angles her jaw, shuffles an inch closer for the kiss. And I kiss her. "See you then," I say. "Be okay. I love you very much."

She says nothing. Her eyes say nothing. Her face is in motion. Her eyes cannot lock with mine.

"You could look out a window," I say. "I'm parked over there. In front of where you come in. You'll see me run out there in the rain. A blue car. The only one by the other side. Near the trees."

"Yes," she says. "Okay. I can look out a window."

"Yes. Good. See you. I'll see you. I'll see you again."

Rain drips steady inside the car, dripping on the cracked dash near the little St. Anthony, plopping on the paper garbage, soaking the seat. The window is down a sliver, fog builds up from the car's defroster blast. I can't see out much and Mother can't see in but I feel her panic, feel her curiosity, the world of her inside out and backwards – can't see rain spewing from the down spouts, gurgling around gutter drains, sliding off the brown brick of her building, beating the third floor windows, the black bars, sliding down steps, over sidewalks. The radio says rain is widespread. Rain falling in Green Bay, the announcer says, falling in Madison – State Street is a river – falling steady over Milwaukee's County stadium, too, where my cousins took me on my thirteenth birthday one last time Gramma went to see Mother. Hammering Hank Aaron came out of his sleep stance, cracked the jumping mean of a Robin Roberts fast ball, I mean Hank exploded that speed pea and stood us straight up off our sky seats – this bead of zip-zipping white slammed into bleacher seats with so much force it shot back onto the field and must have rolled wild a good fifty yards on that perfect grass.

The thunderstorms are widespread, the announcer says, falling rain from La Crosse to Superior, storms in a long line sweeping the state, raining down the shores of Lake Michigan where Mother limped once in hot sand, raining down on the Rambler factory in Kenosha, rain falling at the zoo in Racine, pouring rain falling hard in some places more than others he says with more rain behind us in another storm west of the Mississippi, and rain coming soon to the land of Chicago, drowning Wrigley Field where Mother rode in the bus, rose to the singing, cheered with gusto, ate fat popcorn, sang with everybody, raised her arms when the Cubs hit it good. Raining too in Great Lakes – on Downey VA – raining on Building 131, rain all day and all through the night, expecting more tomorrow the man says, rain accompanied by biblical winds from the tomb of Lazarus, boulder hail, chambers of nuclear thunder, spectacular lightning by Zeus and his twisting mermaid whores.

One radio station blends with another, the other weak through scratches, then strong again, steady, clear as a bell, intelligent, beyond my thoughts to gather in any common sense, understand. I'm going to pound it again and I raise my fist, but then a man begins speaking of his next selection, unique to the world, rather quite amazing he says, his own personal choice of a magnificent sad story about a young woman singing to her father. She sings, he says, about her love for a handsome man and the pain this love has caused her.

"*AriabygiacomopucciniOmiobabbinocarofromtheoperargiannischicchi*"

We should be warned before these events, this cold horror, this soul-soaring, gut trouble – Maria Callas weeping the wail of a wonder woman singing sweet screams through windy rain. How has it come to pass that I've never heard anything like this before?

I'm getting Gramma. Got to. I'll hold her sweet flesh face, tell her again how sorry I am for my sins, tell her to hop in the jitter car because we're going to see her good daughter, Regina. Let's just go, I'll say. I was there. She knew me. She's better. I could tell. You know how some people in these God damn places get better over time?

We'll all go. Grandma and my good wife and my good kids and the Cadillac-me without the stink of rum breath to a nice picnic with Ma, one fine day soon, next week, next month, sooner than next year, a thick shade tree with no nurses, no doctors, no aides, no guards, no secret police with toothpicks, no watchers watching. Hey, we'll relax. Turn on the car radio, crank it to an oldies station. Leave the doors wide. I'll have cash. We'll go shopping, say to the sales clerk, this is my mother, say to the check-out, this is my mother and well she's a grandmother, too. Bring her to a nice family restaurant for milk and pie, say to the waitress, this is my mother and her mother; say to the cashier, this is my mother, and our family, announce her to everyone. Listen up everybody, your attention please, Behold! THIS IS MY MOTHER, say hi, this is her, and when she's a little weary, feeling low, well, isn't she good now really? One royal beauty, goodness with a grin, and I'm her something and something over troubled waters. I'm her something and something melting in the dark, I'm her whiter, better decent shade of pale. And we're getting stronger. You'll see. We'll do this better, get back to the garden, talk about the Lone Ranger and Tonto. We can do this! Look at our lives now, counting clouds, driving off in cheers, radio blaring Bridge Over Troubled Waters. That's it! Sliding like a Silvertone miracle into hit after hit – The Long and Winding Road and Mac Arthur Park, Chug-a-Lug, Chug-a-Lug, The Troggs. One great song after another while she's snug in the seat, giggling, riding low, cooking down those cigarettes, on her way with all of us, a dozen seven-foot mean-ass angels riding outside shotgun on the junk bumpers, on the hot hood, on the scorch-roof, on the hot junk trunk. Step on the gas, this is how you drive the earth ladies and gentlemen. Set your burn-blasters for toast-kill, and if anyone foolish gets in the way on our fast getaway home, don't be afraid no more, please, please dear God, Mommy Regina.

Special Purpose Report: *Regina Jane Van Amber*

It is July 1996, and hot. I am sitting at a conference table six offices and a long hallway deep inside a law firm not far from the Mall of America in Bloomington, Minnesota. Two hours earlier, in the mall's main parking lot, an older woman had tripped and fallen to the pavement. Several, including me, rushed to help. Other than a slight bruise on her right knee and reddened palms, the woman was more embarrassed than hurt, kept looking for the cause of her fall on the parking lot's surface and wondered out loud how it could have happened.

I hadn't thought much about falling before Mother's records arrived. Unthinking people, including several idiot sports celebrities on national television, had made fun of people who had fallen and couldn't get up. I failed to see the humor in that, but it meant nothing personally until I understood how many times Regina had fallen in the VA.

She had been documented as having fallen over one-hundred and ten times – eighty falls during the few years before her death – and those falls, each of those falls, along with the dozens of other outrageous institutional horrors including separate notations of having "one abortion", "lacerated cervix", "has had sex with several men", "has had several children" and "growth on buttocks" – all of that added to the ongoing pressure of doing something about it long after the fact.

Each day since the records had arrived – as Mother's

medical horror unraveled within the pages – I was working toward the revenge of justice, dealing with stubborn VA officials by letter and phone, hoping to arrive at that place the world now so easily and absurdly calls 'closure'.

I might just as well been trying to walk around the moon. Without congressional or public outrage, when it comes to dead psychiatric patients the VA doesn't apologize, rarely compensates the living for medical malpractice on the dead, and never admits guilt.

But because I had appeared on public television in Minneapolis in a nine minute segment, raised my voice once, accused the VA of incompetence and experimentation, filed a Tort claim on behalf of Mother, and asked for an investigation into charges of abuse and neglect, the VA's Central Office, (following political pressure), went to work and pushed Mother's agony into history as far as possible, made me out to appear fanatical for asking questions, and released their 128 page single spaced document titled: "Special Purpose Report: Regina Jane Van Amber."

The VA stated that Regina could not have undergone an abortion in 1977, that she was well beyond child bearing age, didn't have any children in the VA, and that during recent interviews with the examining gynecologist now in private practice in Chicago, he had told them that what was written couldn't have been correct. The special report went on to say that it could not determine why another physician wrote: "Has had sex with several men".

The VA stated that there were some ward files they did not see.

The VA said they hired an independent forensic pathologist who examined the autopsy report, and he had determined there was no prefrontal lobotomy, but that old lobotomy scars could have been missed when her brain was extracted. They went on to say that her name wasn't listed in the surgical log books in Downey as having had a lobotomy, that lobotomies were performed not in Downey anyway, but at the University of Minnesota hospital in Minneapolis, and three other places around the country, and since there was no record of her transfer, she did not have one.

"She did not act like a lobotomy patient," they said, and reminded me, "one should not take things out of context".

The VA said that a lacerated cervix is "normally" lacerated, that her falls were not life threatening, that US government assault reports were missing and they didn't know why, that some former staff could not be located, some did not wish to be interviewed, and the VA has never tolerated patient abuse. The VA said that staff at Downey and Tomah received extensive and comprehensive training on how to care for psychiatric patients.

That staff on the Female Units recalled:

> *baking for patients,*
> *taking them shopping, to dances, parties, fashion shows, cookouts, bingo, bowling and golf,*
> *washing and setting women's hair,*
> *taking them to the beauty parlor,*
> *having a special night for dress-up when all the women would put on make-up and their best dresses,*
> *decorating the units for holidays,*
> *taking patients home for an afternoon or evening to give them a family environment,*
> *that women delivered babies at the Great Lakes Naval Hospital*
> *that Veterans Service Organizations went all out for women on the women's units to make sure they had all the things women wanted or needed, e.g. shampoo, lipstick.*

❖

The VA went on to say that Shock Treatment, Insulin Coma, and Electro-Narcosis was "state of the art" treatment, that during Mother's restraint periods she was given a fifteen-minute break every hour. (So she could put on rouge and tidy up?)

Wet Sheet Packs were not dissimilar to whirlpools and hot tubs in use today, the VA said.

The VA reminded me that Regina had said, "Adolf Hitler is my son."

The VA said they wrote to the pharmaceutical companies regarding her medications but those companies did not respond.

The VA said that while it was true Regina should not have been on anti-Parkinsonian drugs for longer than three months, the three and one half years she was on those drugs were "probably necessary". The VA listed those months when she was overdosed, said it was unfortunate, but insisted those periods did not cause her serious injury.

The VA said my mother was a difficult patient, but commended the family for the number of visits over the years (thirty-nine).

The VA's special report said, "She was treated with love and kindness".

The VA promised to meet with me, to bring the Acting Inspector General, the Chief of Psychiatry, one staffer, sit around a conference table without media or lawyers, discuss what they had written.

The first meeting was canceled because of a government shutdown, the second because of a blizzard in D.C., the third because the VA's Chief of Psychiatry had a hernia operation and "it was too painful for him to travel". The VA's Inspector General told me they had bought the tickets "and everything".

VA officials never did show.

And the VA said it could not explain why several official dozen US Government assault forms were missing. The VA stated that at no time during Mother's thirty-one year hospitalization in their system was she ever assaulted by a staff member. Not once, they said. Never, they said.

Karen Murray had filed suits against the VA through the Tort process for a quarter century. She had lost more than won, made her percentage, seen horrible medical mistakes within the VA's medical system, but had not filed a case on behalf of anyone institutionalized under VA psychiatry.

Before finding Murray, I had contacted eighteen attorneys, none of whom had ever filed a Tort. Because the VA gave me a deadline, I went ahead and filled out the one page document myself, attached fifty pages of personal injuries along with dates and times and witnesses, sent it to the VA's General Counsel in Hines, Illinois, and waited. According to the attorney working for the VA in Downey, my claim was misplaced for a year, then located, then rejected along with a six-month chance for an appeal. I later learned from Murray that I had made a mistake in the place where I was supposed to fill in a "sum certain" amount for wrongful injury, and the way it read now, I wouldn't have gotten a dime even if the VA had accepted the Tort.

Murray had read the Special Purpose Report, looked at the fifty pages of injuries and supporting files, and believed there was a case. I showed her two drawings of a nude woman an artist friend had made. One nude is standing, revealing her back side, and the other her front. Both drawings, from head to toe, were covered with small black dots and marks placed there in pencil, so many dots and marks that the rough physical details on the original drawings could no longer be seen.

Murray looked at the drawings, shook her head slowly.

"We might be able to get past Statute of Limitations," she said. "Especially since the VA was not forthcoming with the records. But you would need to hire several experts to testify, and that could run into a great deal of money. Ten to twenty thousand for starters," she said. "Maybe more."

"Anything else I can try?"

"Not that I know," she said. "Put in a different amount on the claim – millions – send it back to them, see what happens."

"They'll reject it."

"Yes," she said, "but there isn't much else that can be done without experts."

I thanked her for her time, and gathered the stack of papers to leave. On our way out she stopped, turned, and faced me. "I want you to know," she said quietly, "that in the twenty-five years I've been doing this, these are the worse files I've seen. I'm sorry that I can't do more."

Toward the end of the records – at around page 9,000 – is a single sheet listing Mother's personal effects. I had not known of their existence. I wrote to the VA in Tomah asking what had happened and they responded by saying that after three years personal effects are destroyed or given away. I wrote a generic letter to Mother's brothers and sister asking if they knew about her effects. The response from each family was negative.

Uncle Marvin died that summer, and two weeks after the funeral Aunt Digna said she was going through one of his suitcases and found my mother's valuables – rings, necklaces, earrings, and a cigarette case. Some things on the list were missing, but Digna also said that, twelve years earlier, within a few weeks after Mother had died, the VA sent dresses to

REGINA'S RECORD

Marvin and the two had decided the dresses were too stained, too dirty, too ripped to keep. They tossed them in the trash.

I was crushed. I would have hugged her dresses, loved them into a quilt, kept the quilt as a work of family art, passed on the quilt with stories of the woman who once danced in them, fell, breathed, laughed.

I asked my aunt why Marvin hadn't told me about her things, and she said he didn't think I cared about that stuff.

Old age demands more tolerance than it does forgiveness.

I drove two-hundred miles to get my mother's things and on the return trip caressed her cigarette case, her gold wedding set with the fake stone (chipped), her silver necklace, her friendship ring. I slid each ring up to my knuckle joints, put on her gold leaf earrings with pearl centers (for half an hour), drove the Interstate home at just under ten over the speed limit.

Postscript

After locating Mother's original psychiatrist, Dr. Taylor Scorba, I forwarded him copies of records written in his own hand, wondered in writing if I might ask him questions about Mother's case. When he didn't respond, I called him. I asked if the VA had contacted him for their investigation, and he said they had not. He didn't remember my mother, he said, but he did recall "hearing" that some few early lobotomies were performed at Downey and refused further comment. "We must have a bad connection," he said. "And thank you for calling, and good-bye."

After leaving the North Chicago VA, Taylor Scorba became a consulting psychiatrist for Superior Court of the County of Los Angeles and worked at the Sepulveda VA in southern California. Manley Morrison died in 1974. Nothing else is known about Morrison's practice or his life after Downey.

A cousin located and forwarded the California death certificate of Henry James Alle, the man Mother claimed she met on the troop train the day after her discharge and a name she wrote down on the back of my baby pictures as "father". He died in 1964, had never served in the military, and his photograph bears no family resemblance. During the war years, however, he was in San Francisco playing alto sax in the nightclub circuit. He married a widow in 1950, had no children. There is no evidence he was ever in Spokane where I was conceived.

REGINA'S RECORD

❖

According to the Minnesota Department of Human Services, "records on all psychiatric patients discharged from July 1, 1890 through December 31, 1963, in all facilities run by the state, were destroyed".

Mother's records contain over 12,606 individual ward reports (some longer than a page) written by 2,923 nurses, student nurses, and aides. The selections I chose, appear as they were written, not dissimilar to thousands of similar entries. I thought long and hard before changing the names contained in this work, but because mental illness in this country is still considered a primary weakness in human character and a threat to the social fabric, and, because the religion of psychiatry and pharmacology still maintains its financial grip on mental disorders, I didn't want to risk the possibility of ridicule for those family members and others still living.

In the VA's 1995 special report, officials stated at least one obvious truth: "Schizophrenia destroys families".

While I disagree with the VA over numerous points within their report, disturbed by the obvious incompetence revealed within Mother's files, I am grateful officials took the time to investigate her case although I understood from the outset that all government agencies sensitive to outside scrutiny, whether from press or private citizen, protect themselves the best way they can. Lying and misinformation are most certainly part of those methods.

During the year long inquiry, I spoke with the VA's

Inspector General several times, not always in pleasant tones. During our last conversation, a week before the report was released, he stated that what his office had compiled were "just words".

It is the first week in August, 1999. I am sitting in the "Urgent Care" lobby on the main floor of the Minneapolis VA Medical Center, waiting to see a psychiatrist for the first time in thirty-two years. Some have said that this VA is one of the best hospitals in the VA system and the doctors, nurses and staff here have helped thousands of veterans who have come through its doors.

Like many Americans I do not have health insurance and by the time I was done studying Mother's records, going through the VA's investigation of her ordeal, and trying to finish this book, it felt like my entire body had been beaten with a spiked broom handle. My energy was sapped. The simplest things took concentrated effort. I had trouble getting out of bed and little stamina for much of anything after that. I wondered if a psychiatrist might make some suggestions and I could get on with living. I also was curious whether or not I might sense that same risk I often felt dealing with government sponsored psychiatry .

Fools never learn.

A few minutes after I had given a hospital intake-worker basic information which would qualify me for VA care, she called me back to the counter where another clerk wondered out loud why the computer would not allow him to access my files. He referred to them as "case sensitive" and added, "I've only known two reasons that this could happen. For a file to be secure like this, a person would either have to be in the witness protection program or a former or current VA employee".

"None of those," I said. "Unless it's the initials of my last name or something weird like that." He chuckled, then looked at my name. "Oh, I get it. V-A!"

Another clerk joined the first two, mentioned the need to make a phone call, but would let me know in a few minutes what they came up with, and why they couldn't access my military records without permission.

I went back to my seat and waited, aware of the curious glances. The three were unsure, I suppose, about what to make of my situation, careful not to make it obvious.

While they try to straighten matters out, I take out a new brass coin from my pocket and began rubbing it between thumb and forefinger. It's about the size of a half-dollar. On one side of this wonderful coin is the Prayer for Serenity. On the flip side is the number 25 in Roman numerals. The outer edge of this coin has the words: "To Thine Own Self Be True." The people who gave me this coin, along with a birthday cake the week before, say that I am an inspiration to them and my good wife is a saint for putting up with me, my good children are lucky to have me as their father and my little granddaughters are cute as a bug's ear. I have not had a drink for more than twenty-four years. One man in this group of good friends is a retired teacher. He spoke through tears – said that if it weren't for me he'd be utterly lost or at least deep in the woods.

One woman, a stay-at-home mom, said that because of her own imperfections and the constant committee in her head, she used to be scared of me, but that was no longer true and that I am like a brother to her and she loves me and my family. One man who rides a Harley looked at me and in a loud voice said this: "I have never told any man, including my old man, that I loved him, and I don't intend to ever say this again, but I love you." The Harley man's wife, who rides the big Harley with him, said she thought I was a God damn bona fide miracle in the flesh and the sickest son-of-a-bitch she ever knew and loved, and if I can make it to twenty-five years without joy juice, by God anybody can. A man who is learning to read and write wept because he said he couldn't find the words. Another man, a professor at a nearby university, said he loved this new way of life and he was glad that I was in it with him.

I tell these friends that I have no idea what will happen tomorrow, but I still have quite a lot of work to do and I need all the help I can get. And I do.

As I am rubbing this coin, thinking about recent past events, the VA clerk, who promised to let me know about what he found out from the computer mix-up, approached me, said that all they needed to know in the first place, really, was if my discharge was honorable. And it was. That I qualified for help and everything was all right. Then he retreated a little, turned to leave, hesitated, and faced me again, grinning. "For what it's worth about what's on the computer, you, or maybe one of your relatives, must have given the VA hell about something once. Whatever it was, don't worry about it."

There may well be another reason my files had restricted access. The VA is protecting my status as a former patient in order to protect itself from any legal action should my files fall into the wrong hands.

Sometime later I followed a psychiatric nurse into a room where the questions began. I'd heard them before, of course, tweaked and re-worded over and over in different ways. *"Ever have any unusual telephone conversations? Ever wanted to kill someone? Ever had suicidal thoughts? What is the date today? (I made sure I knew it just in case) How much coffee do you drink? How much do you smoke? Do you have any weapons on you now? Do you own any weapons? Ever been in jail? Ever been hospitalized for mental illness? Ever been on medications? Ever been arrested for DUI? Ever heard voices? Anyone in your family mentally ill?"*

REGINA'S RECORD

After a few minutes, the nurse escorts me into a little room where a man playing his part as this handsome, intelligent, well-groomed, middle-age board certified VA psychiatrist with frameless glasses introduces himself and asks me to sit down. After a brief discussion about the possibilities of depression and what might be done about it, he suggested the nurse make an appointment for me to start therapy sessions in a week. He said it would be a good idea for me to see a psychiatrist again regarding the possibility of medications. "In the last five years there's been a lot of new advanced medications without many side-effects," he said. "Something to think about for later."

And finally, in a kind but somewhat solicitous tone, he began the questions again, tweaked again, disguised by his rearrangement of words.

> *"Do you feel as if the wolf is at your door,"* he asked.
> *"Would you just like to fall asleep and not wake up?*
> *Ever have what you would consider unusual telephone conversations?*
> *Ever wanted to really just kill someone?*
> *Ever had suicidal thoughts?*
> *Ever thought of ways to kill yourself? The method?*
> *What is today's date?*
> *Do you have any weapons on you now?*
> *Ever been in the hoosegow?*
> *Ever been hospitalized for mental illness?*
> *Ever had thoughts telling you what to do or what to write?*
> *Ever been on medications?*
> *Ever been picked up for DUI?*
> *Ever heard voices?*

Ever count things?
Where are we now?
What was your mother's mental illness?
How long was she in the VA? Did you know her?
Did you visit her? Did she know you?
Who raised you?"

It's easy to find my car in the parking lot. Six hours earlier it took me five minutes to get a spot. And I did have this thought about leaving the engine running just in case I needed to make an exit, but the exit wouldn't have been all that quick. My legs hurt and I'm sluggish and it was an absurd idea because by now the engine would've run out of gas, and the battery would have died, so it was a good thing I didn't.

My plan was to stop for a bite to eat on the drive south. But instead of driving home, I changed my mind, decided on another destination, drove west on I-94 for two and a half hours and finally turned off at my old home town exit to a seven mile stretch south before turning east on that last road I saw my mother when I was a child. The landscape hasn't changed much, paved roads, a few new signs, a satellite dish or two on lawns near the few small farms along the two-mile stretch. I made another turn south toward Maple Lake, spotted the north side of the old creamery house, stopped near the ditch not far from the mailbox. From where I stood it didn't look like anyone lived in Ted's old place anymore. The last owner had planted pine trees in the yard, blocking much of the view to the old porch kitchen. The creamery table is gone, but I know where it is. The woman who bought the place from old Ted wanted to get rid of it, hired some local men who came with a dump truck and a backhoe. They attached a chain around its belly, tried lifting it off its foundation, but it wouldn't budge so they rammed it with the truck to push it over or break it in two, and when that didn't work, dropped the backhoe's bucket on the table to smash it into chunks. After half an hour of hacking at the thing, the woman said that the cement didn't show as much as a crack. There was talk of dynamite, but instead the men dug a hole deep around the table's base, toppled the thing over, and covered it with dirt.

I danced for Mother on that table.

The garden plot is gone, still a garden in one way, connected to the farmer's larger field.

On my keyring are mother's dog tags from World War II along with her golden service medal given to each veteran who served during that war. It is sunset over the slough, and sounds of the night begin to rise as the prelude to an orchestral event that has gone on for centuries. The Sioux who once lived here heard it, and my mother heard it, and my grandparents heard it, and Ted heard it, and I heard it. I slip one dog tag off the ring, take the precious medal out of its holder, and fling both toward a row of beans near what once was the path that led from the ditch to the little house.

In a couple days, when I feel a little stronger and my mind clears and my emotions level out, I'll start looking for work again. Sometime tomorrow or the next day I'll call and cancel the appointment with VA therapists. No need to explain. Call, cancel, thank you, goodbye, hang up. They can keep their asterisk on my file and let it ride into cyberspace.

When I get back home, if the "wolf" the psychiatrist talked about comes to the door, I'll have no reason not to invite him in. Wolves, I'm told, are much more fearful than dangerous. Besides, the wolf has been in my life before, lots of times, and I keep thinking about how we're beginning to get used to one another after all these years.

I steer the car past the mailbox and into the old driveway, back out, drive north to the longer road and turn west. No reason or need to come this way again, look back over the north field toward the garden and the house as I had done so many times as a child.

Skeeter Davis is on the radio, loud. Turned it off.

> *You God of garden and stone and weed and plant, bless my family and the people in my heart. You Mother God, bless my good aunts and uncles and their good children, my cousins, and their good children. O God, bless my mother who suffered on this earth. You Lord of light and air, bless my good wife and our good children and our good grandchildren. May God bless old Ted, a hermit who was kind to me. May God and the Angels bless the Lone Ranger and Tonto, and bless the great Sioux who once dwelt under these heavens and had to leave. You God of goodness, bless the night and the day, and all of us everywhere who are just now learning to live and love, to laugh and weep.*

And He [Jesus] said to the paralytic, "I say to you, rise, take up your pallet and go home."
Gospel According to Mark 2:11

ACKNOWLEDGEMENTS

This work would not have been possible without the patient detachment of my wife, Mary, and the encouragement and skill of other writers, poets, researchers, educators, college students, politicians, reporters, family members, VA officials and nurses, and friends who have taken considerable risks of their own on my behalf.

For as long as I live I will never know how to adequately thank Roger Sheffer who came to my rescue many, many times with daily guidance, support and encouragement.

Sincere thanks to my son, Jon, who painstakingly designed an impressive cover jacket that actually said it all, without any need for words.

Thanks also to Jane Saunders for her patience with the numerous checking and rechecking of the manuscript.

Finally, it seems fitting that through fate, faith and the new frontier called Cyberspace, Regina's Record found a home in an unlikely place with an uncommon author, editor and publisher. Heartfelt thanks to Elaine Sihera, without whose perseverance and vision, and the good work of her staff in Marlow, my mother's story, and mine (along with perhaps countless others who have suffered in silence behind the closed walls of an institution), would remain no more than a fading whisper on the final landscape of institutional horror and indifference during the latter half of the twentieth century.

APPENDIX: VA Policy References

It is impossible to list all the sources quoted from the thousands of documents used, but the following provides a flavour for further information:

* Department of Medicine and Surgery, G-1, M-2, Part X, Program Guide, Psychiatry and Neurology Service, March 15, 1955.

* Department of Medicine and Surgery, G-2, M-2, Part X, Program Guide, Psychiatry and Neurology Service, May 2, 1955.

* Department of Medicine and Surgery, G-4, M-2, Part X, Program Guide, Psychiatry and Neurology Service, July 1, 1955.

* Department of Medicine and Surgery, M-2, Part X, Professional Services, Psychiatry and Neurology Service, November 4, 1955.

* Department of Medicine and Surgery, G-6, M-2, Part X, Program Guide, Psychiatry and Neurology Service, November 15, 1955.

* Department of Medicine and Surgery, G-8, M-2, Part X, Program Guide, Psychiatry and Neurology Service, April 9, 1956.

* Department of Medicine and Surgery, G-13, M-2, Part X, Program Guide, Mental Health and Behavioral Sciences Services, Inpatient Guide for Psychiatry, December 15, 1977.

* Department of Medicine and Surgery, G-14, M-2, Part X, Program Guide, Mental Health and Behavioral Sciences Services, Antischizophrenic Drug Use, February 15, 1978.

* Department of Medicine and Surgery, G-15, M-2, Part X, Program Guide, Mental Health and Behavioral Sciences Services, Management of the Violent and Suicidal Patient, March 13, 1978.

* Department of Medicine and Surgery, G-16, M-2, Part X, Guidelines for the Use of Antidepressant Drugs Program Guide, Mental Health and Behavioral Sciences Service, December 30, 1980.

* Department of Medicine and Surgery, M-2, Part XIV, Surgical Service, November 20, 1955, and subsequent relevant changes including, Change 19, January 31, 1973, Change 26, December 23, 1976, and Change 29, August 27, 1982.

* Department of Medicine and Surgery, M-2, Part X, Psychiatry and Neurology Service, November 4, 1955, and revision April 23, 1965 and relevant change, Change 2, June 23, 1967.

* Department of Medicine and Surgery, M-2, Part I, Chapter 23, Change 66, Informed Consent, August 27, 1982.

* Veterans Administration Manual, MP-1, Part I, Chapter 23, VA Investigation Policy, October 25, 1954, Change 1, November 9, 1967, Change 2, April 12, 1967, Change 3, November 12, 1973, and Department of Medicine and Surgery Supplements Change 1, April 3, 1955, Change 3, June 27, 1956, Change 6, August 23, 1957, Change 22, May 18, 1966, Change 29, August 1, 1972, and Change 38, 1982.

* Technical Bulletin 10-500, Electric Shock Therapy, November 5, 1947.

* Technical Bulletin 10A-243, Assault Upon, Injury to, Unusual Death and Elopement of Beneficiaries, November 7, 1950.

* Technical Bulletin 10-42, Shock Therapies of the Psychoses, February 18, 1948.

* Technical Bulletin 10-501, Insulin Shock Therapy in Schizophrenia, April 16, 1948.

* Technical Bulletin 10A-243, Assault Upon, Injury to, Unusual Death and Elopement of Beneficiaries, November 7, 1950.

* Technical Bulletin 10-42, Shock Therapies of the Psychoses, February 18, 1948.

* Technical Bulletin 10-501, Insulin Shock Therapy in Schizophrenia, April 16, 1948.

* Technical Bulletin 10A-243, Assault Upon, Injury to, Unusual Death and Elopement of Beneficiaries, November 7, 1950.

* Technical Bulletin 10A-272, Consent for Surgical Operations and Electric and Insulin Shock Therapy, July 9, 1951.

REGINA'S RECORD

* Circular 10-64-136, Prior Consent of Patients to Participate in a Study of or the Use of Investigational Drugs, July 6, 1964.

* Circular 10-67-117, Prior Consent of Patients to Participate in the Use of Drugs and/or Procedures for Investigational Purposes, June 2, 1967.

* Circular 10-68-129, Admission of Women Veterans to VA and Non-VA Hospitals, July 12, 1968.

* Circular 10-72-246, Surgery for Abnormal Behavior (Psychosurgery), October 20, 1972.

* Circular 10-76-37, Psychiatric Patients Under Involuntary Commitment in VA Hospitals, March 8, 1976.

Book Reference

Psychosurgery, Freeman & Watts, 2nd Ed. 1950, Charles C. Thomas, Pub. Springfield, Ill.